Praise for *Your Body Believes Every Word You Say*

"Barbara does an enlightening and entertaining job of illustrating how the words and images we use in our daily expression of life can be metaphors for our health status. More importantly, she shows how we can change the course of illness and dysfunction by becoming more aware of, and choosing more carefully, those words and images. Perhaps the most significant 'discovery' of the late twentieth century is the realization that our attitudes and beliefs shape our perceptions and our lives, and that we can become aware of and change these perceptions, producing profound effects on the physical body. Cheers to Barbara for a helpful and empowering book!"
> —Emmett E. Miller, M.D., Medical Director, Cancer Support and Education Center; Author, *Deep Healing: The Essence of Mind/Body Medicine*

"I work with individuals dealing with fibromyalgia, chronic pain syndrome, and chronic fatigue. This book had such a great impact on me personally that I brought Barbara Levine's ideas into my professional life. By using examples and illustrations from her works, I have been able to show my patients dramatic similarities between their use of certain phrases and statements and their clinical diagnosis, or their most common complaints. Many of my patients have been able to move out of patterns that have been keeping them 'stuck,' and into a new reality. Instead of feeling like a victim, these individuals now have the ability to take control of their own healing. I thank her for sharing her story and touching so many lives."
> —Cindy Hodges, Occupational Therapist; owner, A/V Health Services, Inc.

"I was deeply moved by Barbara Levine's personal story. It is obvious that she is a woman of great courage and strength and that she has harnessed these qualities well."
> —Kitty Dukakis, Former First Lady, State of Massachusetts

"I think you have certainly captured a very important aspect of health and self-help in your book."
> —Charles B. Inlander, President, People's Medical Society

"Thank you for your clarity, persistence and vision. Your lessons will be an inspiration to our patients."
> —Barry S. Taylor, N.D., New England Family Health Center

"The self-help exercises alone make the book worth owning. Thank you for an important book."
> —Ginny Fickel, Director, Acoustic Neuroma Association

"We believe that your book would be helpful to many NPF Members."
> —Glennis McNeal, National Psoriasis Foundation

"Not only is it clearly written and a delight for a critical, ex-medical editor to read, but it contains a wealth of practical ideas for healing and the self-help directions for carrying them out."
> —Robert A. Barrett, Ph.D.

"I am certainly going to use your book to improve my own life *and* to explain your wonderful message to my clients and students all over India."
—Dr. Aminuddin Khan, Hyderabad, India

"I really think a second reading of any book confirms whatever thoughts you had the first time and triggers new ones. This happened to me as I just finished rereading your book. I have some wonderful reactions to it the second time."
—Florence Yudkin, Israel

"I can tell you that not only my heart has healed as a result of me reading your book—many other aspects of my body have as well. I'm enjoying better health than before and I'm also happier. So all in all, you've been a great catalyst in my life."
—Gudrun Bergman, Publisher, Iceland

"I enjoyed your book tremendously but wish it would have been available earlier. I had encephalitis and am left with serious neurologic and vestibular problems. I highly recommend it as 'must reading' for every person or family with a chronic illness. Additionally I think it would be most useful for religious leaders who counsel people with health problems, psychologists, psychiatrists and all health care personnel. I intend to recommend it in two of my medical columns. Do write another book. You have great talent, insight and a wonder-fully compassionate writing ability."
—Dr. Susan L. Engel-Arieli, M.D.

"Barbara's very spirit-field says "gifted of God." One encounters her as a divine encounter, a rare blend of this world and this world transcended."
—Dr. Cecil L. "Chip" Murray, Senior Minister, First African Methodist Episcopal Church of Los Angeles

"I'm in the middle of re-reading your book. Love it! Like some other things, its better the second time around."
—Phil Kavanaugh, M.D., Author, *Magnificent Addiction*

"Delighted to be associated in any way with your wonderful book. I think the message of hope and understanding you give should be shouted from the roof tops."
—Jackie Rose, Founder and Director, Association of Retired Persons, U.K.

"Barbara's ability in communications shines forth in her book as she puts together 15 years of research and amazing discoveries to support the title. If you ever had doubts before about how your words and thoughts affect your body, you won't after reading this book.
—Geraldine M. Paulette Bennett, Author, *Opening the Door to Your Inner Self*

"An inspiring read and reinforced for me the power of the mind over the body and the importance of the language we use. Consequently, it will be a valuable addition to our Health Science Library which is used by our staff and many students."
—Marie A. Turbie, Vice President, Patient Care Services, St. Vincent's Medical Care Center, Bridgeport CT

Your Body Believes Every Word You Say

by

Barbara Hoberman Levine

WordsWork Press
An Imprint of R. B. Luce Publishing
Fairfield, Connecticut
USA

Words Work Press
An Imprint of R.B. Luce Publishing
2490 Black Rock Turnpike, #342
Fairfield, CT 06825
Please contact the publisher for a free catalog.
Phone: **203/372-0300**
Fax: **203/374-4766**
www.wordsworkpress.com

IMPORTANT NOTE TO READERS:

The suggestions in this book for personal healing and growth are not meant to substitute for the advice of a licensed professional such as a medical doctor or psychiatrist. It is essential to consult such a professional in the case of any physical or mental symptoms. The publishers and author expressly disclaim any liability for injuries resulting from use by readers of the methods contained herein.

Library of Congress Cataloging-in-Publication Data
Levine, Barbara Hoberman.
    Your body believes every word you say: the language of the
BodyMind connection / by Barbara Hoberman Levine. -- 2nd. ed.
     p. cm.
    Includes biographical references and index.
    ISBN 0-88331-219-0 (trade paper) — ISBN 0-88331-217-4 (hardcover)
    1. Health. 2. Mind and body. 3. Emotions--Health aspects. 4.
Sick--Language. I. Title.
RA776.L646 2000
616'.001'9--dc21   99-022896
                                 CIP

Edited by Marcia Yudkin
Book design by Dianne Schilling
Cover design by Miggs Burroughs
Printing by Baker Johnson, Inc.
Printed in the USA
Second Edition

*This book is joyously dedicated to my family
for loving me unconditionally, through thick and thin,
no matter what I said or did.*

*To my wonderful husband, Harold Levine;
To my terrific sister, Arlene Hoberman Kyler;
To my dear children,
Jennifer, Steven, and Kenneth;*

*To Jennifer's husband Scott French
and
To Kenneth's wife, Linda Rozans, and their children,
my precious granddaughters, Rachel Anne Levine,
and Miriam Sarah Levine.*

Thoughts

Watch your thoughts; they become words.
Watch your words; they become actions
Watch your actions; they become habits.
Watch your habits; they become character.
Watch your character; for it becomes your destiny.

—Unknown

Foreword

Barbara H. Levine's book stayed with me long after I read it. As a writer with a chronic immune disorder, I have read many books about healing, and spiritual tomes galore. My condition affected my walking, among other things, for nine years. I had inklings that perhaps my condition was symbolic in a sense—trouble walking through life; difficulty "standing up" for myself, and *Your Body Believes Every Word You Say* expanded my understanding of the role played by thought and language in this phenomenon.

In clear yet absorbing prose, Barbara H. Levine explores how her own words, ideas and beliefs had an impact on her health. However, she clearly avoids the blame game played by some alternative healing mavens, a guilt by commission or omission kind of suggestion—in other words, you could heal yourself, so if you're not healed, you're not doing it right. Levine gently deals with this issue and moves on to make me a believer in just what her title so aptly proclaims.

Two years passed after I read the book, and when the time was right, I plucked it off my shelf and reread it—something I often plan with good books, but rarely do. The book was packed with new insights for me, and was just as fresh and interesting the second time around.

Since reading it, I have "caught" myself many times, as I did just last week, when I tripped, acquiring a hairline fracture in my left arm. I heard myself telling a friend that my arm was "killing" me, and made an immediate correction. "It's not killing me," I said. "It just hurts." Why add unnecessary drama, and give my arm's pain power? That's what this book is about, for me, the power of awareness, something anyone can benefit from, whether they are just dealing with everyday challenges or special health issues.

—Judith Wershil

Judith Wershil is a writer, counselor and interfaith minister. She has written for the New York Times and Gannett newspapers among many others.

Acknowledgments

So many people supported me in writing both the original and the 2nd edition of this book. You have my thanks even if I don't mention your name. I love you all and wish you the best.

Special thanks to W.C. Ellerbroek, M.D., now deceased, whose ideas sparked my own and who so generously shared his thoughts with me. Special thanks and big hugs to Bernie Siegel, M.D., and Emmett Miller, M.D., both of whom went out of their way to encourage me from the earliest stages of my work on this book during the first edition and who continue to support and encourage me, even now. Their belief in me helped me to believe in myself and encouraged me to ask for help from the rest of the health community.

Thanks for editorial contributions: from M.D.s Harry Brown, David Bushell, Steve Hirshorn, Steven Kunkes, Bob Lang, Ron Levin, Larry Novik, Vincent Scavo, Robban Sica, Montague Ullman and nurse Judy Chessin; from dentists Randy Neichen and Mark Breiner; from chiropractors Robert Marshall, and Jacqueline Ruzga; from naturopaths Larry Caprio and Marvin Schweitzer; from optometrist Carl Gruning, physicist Buryl Payne and pastoral counselor Bari Dworkin; from therapists Debbie Blair, Julia Bondi, Eric Esselstyn, Denny Cooper & Sarah Gewanter, Jack Henry, Alice Katz, Ananda Saha, Ted Smith, Roberta Tager, Dorothy Thau and Linda Zelizer.

In addition to those health professionals already mentioned, thanks to Drs. Abrams, Baker, Bekoff, Burd, Brown; Cohen, Dogali, Epstein, Gill, Hankin, Hu, Kauders, Rich Levin, Levy, Lipow, Luck, McAleer, Rago, Reichgut, Rosa, Sachs, Sasaki, Schiff, K. Siegel, Jeff Small and Peter Small for unswerving support during and since the years of my research. Special thanks to friends, teachers and massage therapists Jeanne Cheney, Lydia Dixon, Clare Mastromonaco and Janice Schwartz.

Thanks to graduate school teachers Ruth Gonchar Brennan, Joe Cahalan, Ted Cheney, Jim Keenan, Jackie Rinaldi and Barry Tarshis, who, among others, nurtured my writing and communications skills.

To writer friends and others for suggested improvements and writing support during the first or second edition: Judy Berkun, Jacquie Bishop, Ralph Carruthers, Chuck Cordova, Barry Diamond, Nadine Fauerbach, Charlie Fried, Liz Goldner, George Markley, Michael Mesmer, Michael Millman, Nancy Nehlsen, Joyce Saltman, Howie Sann, Naomi Schaffer and Melissa Schnirring. To Judy Glaser for the "human as instrument" analogy; to Susan Flaster and to Myrin Borysenko, whose good words came when I needed them most; to Marilyn Ferguson for being a role model and sharing the information in *Brain/Mind Bulletin*.

To my first agent, Adele Leone, for introducing me to then Aslan Publishers Brenda Plowman and Dawson Church. They were the best publishers a first-time author could have and remain dear friends though they no longer own Aslan. My husband, Hal, and I do. To Jenny D'Angelo for sending love copy-editing the first edition. To Michael Karpilow for proving that I am photogenic. To Sandy Satterwhite, my agent and friend, whose encouragement was key to my completing this new edition of the book.

Major credit goes to my editors. Marcia Yudkin, dear friend and mentor, guided and encouraged me through every revision prior to the first edition. Her belief in me and her sensitivity to the material was crucial. Dawson Church took over before the first edition came out and pushed and prodded me, ever so gently, until finally we both knew we had the book we wanted. Judy Tompkins pressed me to write this updated edition after a long bout of procrastination. Marcia Yudkin also lovingly edited this new edition.

Special thanks and praise to my new friend and colleague Dianne Schilling for designing this edition and making sure I stayed on time and on target. Thanks to both Dianne and Marcia for not allowing my publisher's hat to be superseded by my author's hat thus keeping the book focused on what mattered. Thanks to Miggs Burroughs for creating a new cover that surpassed my expectations and for allowing me into his studio for more hands-on work in the creation.

For inspiration and information thanks to John Bear, Stewart Emery, Werner Erhard, John Graham, Henry Reed and John-Roger. To Gene and Eva Graf, Baba Muktananda (deceased), Gurumayi Chidvilasananda, Acharya Sushil Kumar Muni Ji (deceased), Rabbi Arnold Sher, Grace 'n Vessels of Christ, Kenneth Copeland and my many prayer partners for spiritual sustenance, information, and growth prior to publication of the first edition. I acknowledge my gratitude to all my former teachers and students from whom I learned so much.

After publication of the first edition, I turned to Judaism, the faith of my parents. My newfound interest profoundly affected me and informed my writing in this revised and expanded edition. I wish to thank everyone associated with Congregation B'nai Israel in Bridge-port—it would be impossible to mention all those who have influenced me. On the other hand you know who you are—especially those of you who have become personal friends.

Special thanks to the professional, janitorial, security and office staffs; to the regulars who worship together each weekend bringing music and prayer to nurture my soul; to those with whom I study Torah each week; to the members of our religious practices committee and the monthly Rosh Chodesh group each of whom encouraged me in their own way even when they didn't know that was what they were doing.

Thanks to Bnai Israel educators Bob and Marsha Gillette, Ira Wise, Elaine Chetrit and especially Ariela Ben Dor who recognized a soul connection and encouraged the tiny spark to ignite as she taught me to read Hebrew; to Cantor Ray Gilbert who believed I could do it and taught me to chant the prayers and Torah for my Bat Mitzvah in 1993.

Thanks to Cantor Sheri Blum who weekly gives voice to my inner yearnings. She makes the sounds that I feel inside but have no way to express. Her joyfulness and music inspires us all. Thanks to Rabbi Jim Prosnit, who was and continues to be my guide and teacher along the Torah Path, to Rabbinic Intern Ruth Zlotnick and to local Rabbis Waldman, Baum, Stein and Yasgur who welcome me even though I am from a different congregation.

To author Rabbis Steven Rosman and Ted Falcon, my dear friends and boosters who encouraged and supported me and had faith in my abilities even when my faith seemed to lag; to the Jewish renewal leaders and spiritual teachers on the P'nai-Or rabbinical e-mail list especially—Libby Bottero for so many helpful words, Gideon Weisz for Abracadabra, Goldie Milgram and Dr. Barry Bub for sharing a special journey and more, and Linda Zweig for her teaching that "the flame of the universe is fueled by every one of us."

To all the wonderful authors who travel this journey with Aslan Publishing and WordsWork Press; to our attorney Alan Neigher; to Jimmy Twyman the "Peace Troubador and Emissary Of Light" who brought so much to our lives; to mentor Vivian Bradbury, printer Wayne Johnson and our public relations guru Michelle Rathman for their special expertise; to the sales reps and any others who brought this book to market and to the reader's attention. Especial thanks to the readers of the first edition who recommended and endorsed the book—many wrote me encouraging or inspiring letters. We've included just a few in these pages.

To all my Estrin and Hoberman cousins who love unconditionally and to Diane & Rolland French; To old friends for being there when I needed them: Gemma Abboud, Jim Bacik, Terry Caprio, Ruth Casl, Gail Cohen, Elly Davidson, Betty Hauptman, Meryl Kessler, Barbara Lachs, Irma Lesser, Ruth and Jack Levine, Debby Masone, John & Jane Mather, Lois O'Brien, Tony Storace, Ray Tata, Mary and John Steinmetz, John Moretti, Ruth and Sarn Perelson, Judi and David Rosner, Lele, Clark and Claudia Stephens, Jean Swilling and Jo Willard.

To Helen and Roy Diton, Eileen & Mike Glassman, Linda Singer, and all the 2402 Brooklyn families; to Swatonah campmates, to alumni of Seth Low, Lafayette, CCNY/Baruch and Fairfield University Graduate School of Communication where this book was conceived.

Special thanks to my parents, Abraham and Evelyn Hoberman, (now deceased), for giving birth to me and my sister and nurturing us through the early years. To Arlene and Jerry Kyler, and David and Jackie Levine, for steadfast love and loyalty in good times and bad. To Harold Levine for being everything I wanted and needed in a husband—you continue to surprise and amaze me almost every day. To my children and grandchildren, nieces and nephews for their love, their support and the lessons taught; to the loving G!d who dwells within and without and the Angels who watch over me, protect me, and show me the way to go and The Path to follow.

As I complete these final steps in the second edition, new names keep emerging to be thanked. I am reminded anew that we are all interconnected and that even very limited interactions can have a profound effect.

Many Blessings,
Barbara Hoberman Levine
22 Tevet 5760

Contents

Self-Help Experiences

If at first you don't succeed, try, try, again.

I can complain because a rose bush has thorns or rejoice because a thorn bush has roses.

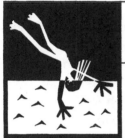 # Chapter 1

How I Came to Write This Book

Who would have guessed that having a brain tumor would be the most beneficial, life saving adventure of my life? If anyone had told me the day would come when I would give thanks for having a brain tumor, I would have said, "You're crazy." If anyone had told me back in 1970 that 25 years later I would be thanking God for the gift of a brain tumor, I would have thought "You have rocks in your head."

Nevertheless, it's true! I would not even have this wonderful, exciting, fulfilling life now except for the fact that for many years I lived with, learned from, and wrote about this awesome brain tumor experience. And I do thank God for the ability to use this seemingly adverse event as a positive one rather than as a tragedy. Make no mistake, going through it wasn't pleasant. There were days when I wallowed in despair, anger and self-pity. I was a master of self-pity. Yet I do give thanks for the many blessings I received from learning, healing and growing along with the tumor, even as I pray for further improvement.

The Brain Tumor: My Growth

The ideas in this book arose from the life-changing experience that seemed to begin in 1970 with the birth of my third child, Jennifer. But looking back, I see the experience actually began in 1966 when I became an adult orphan. Both my parents died, in their early fifties of heart disease, 10 months apart. This mind-boggling event came as an enormous shock. I became fearful and depressed, but I wasn't adept at handling or understanding my feelings at that time. Then, after Jennifer's birth, I thought I was finally perfectly happy. But the stress of the previous four years had affected me physically as well as emotionally.

I developed a weakness in my voice and could barely talk above a whisper. Doctors told me my left vocal cord was paralyzed, but they didn't know why. I was 32 years old. The pain I suffered searching for a diagnosis was almost unbearable, making me feel even sicker. Every test came back negative. A virus was blamed, when no one could find another cause. After that I lived in terror — afraid of getting sicker, afraid of taking more medical tests, not even sure I would live. A year later I became deaf in my left ear. Doctors again blamed a virus.

At that time, I was fat, a heavy smoker, and in poor physical condition. Having a paralyzed left vocal cord and a deaf left ear actually helped push me in the *right* direction. I realized I needed to find a way to live longer and healthier, so I could be with my two sons and my new daughter as they grew into adulthood. Living to see my children grow up was very important to me, motivating me to survive — no matter what.

I began to live one day at a time, relieving my fear whenever possible by enjoying some of the good things in my life — a nice family, good friends, and a comfortable home. After a year, my voice began to improve somewhat, even though the paralysis and deafness remained. My fear became more bearable when I focused on my newly-found-life-purpose, which was to perfect my ability to think for myself and help others to do the same. Working for women's rights, helping women become more self-aware and learning how to heal myself were key elements in this quest.

My real growth began when I learned to live each day more fully — because I didn't know how much time I had left. As I successfully lived through each day, I started to believe that I might live long enough to see my children grow up. "One day at a time" became a guiding principle in my life.

Beginning to Heal

For the next four years, my doctors and I blamed my debilitating physical symptoms on viruses, because the need to have a reason was so strong. I didn't have any further tests until 1974 when — after getting myself in shape mentally and physically — I felt I was ready to handle anything that came up. I remember prophetically thinking, "Even if I need brain surgery I can handle it now." After more tests, I finally received an accurate diagnosis. I had a rare, slow-growing, non-malignant tumor. A biopsy, done through my left ear proved that I had *a growth in my head*.

No tumor had been found in 1970 (this was before CAT scans) but my growth began then — physically, mentally, emotionally, and spiritually. Notice the multiple meanings of the word *growth*. At that time, in 1974, a neurosurgeon told me he considered the tumor inoperable, as the potential for brain damage from surgery was too great. The tumor was wrapped around several nerves at the point where they exited my brain, next to the brain stem. It was putting pressure on the cranial nerves, affecting my speech and hearing. But thankfully the tumor was benign, slow-growing, and small enough for me to live with. It was a partial relief, as well as unsettling, to finally know the truth.

After this diagnosis, the one big question was how to heal myself, or at least prevent the tumor from growing to life-threatening proportions. The medical community didn't offer much help beyond one doctor's recommendation to "maybe try radiation treatment." He didn't sound at all convinced that that therapy would help. So I declined, believing that radiation would harm me more than help me. Given what I have learned since then, I know I made the correct decision. *If we believe that a treatment will harm us, there's a good chance that it will.*

On the other hand, because I believed that doctors had no real help to offer me, I didn't look further within the medical community. I didn't follow up, in any way, on the recommendation to try radiation treatment. I didn't even ask for more information.

Years after publication of the first edition of this book in 1991, I learned about an effective radiation technique called Stereotactic Radiosurgery. I've been told that this technique was available, in a cruder form, back in 1974. Less intrusive than brain surgery, it successfully slows growth in malignant and benign tumors and sometimes even shrinks the tumor.

I still feel I made the right decision for my long-term growth. But now and in the future, I am committed to being open-minded. I check out any, and all, treatments. I also recognize that the patient needs to be pro-active and do his or her own research of the mainstream medical literature. Today the Internet is making researching and networking for medical information much easier and more rewarding. Recently on the Net, I had the opportunity to advise a woman for whom radiation therapy was recommended. Her concerns and resistance were similar to my own. After hearing what I had to say , she was willing to take advantage of the opportunity to check out the treatment that I was ignorant about. Back in 1974, my beliefs blocked me from checking further into radiation therapy.

Instead I began using holistic healing techniques working on the physical, mental, emotional & spiritual level. I explored diet, exercise, massage, chiropractic, Rolfing, prayer, meditation, Reiki, polarity, and several other energy healing modalities. You name it, I probably tried it. For a year, I fasted one day a week on fresh juices, detoxifying my body and improving my health enormously.

When years passed with no new symptoms — I ignored little signs — I told myself I was healed. I thought, "The tumor probably dissolved when I fasted." I didn't have a CAT scan after they became available, perhaps preferring ignorant bliss over the news of an inoperable growth. When a doctor suggested I take X-rays to check the status of the tumor, I practically turned and ran. What good would it do me to know? To get through each day, I needed to believe it was gone. I believed in my positive inner growth. I was healthy and growing stronger mentally, emotionally and spiritually.

In addition to self-healing, my life revolved around my family and helping others in a variety of ways. I began teaching courses for women about women. Later, as my studies and personal growth continued, I taught Communication, Meditation, Metaphysics, and Holistic Health courses to both men and women.

In 1971, as president of the Western Connecticut National Organization for Women (NOW) chapter, I ran a Women's Sexuality Conference. After studying for a non-academic Metaphysical Science degree (M.Sc.), I did private counseling. The form of my work has often changed, but the underlying thread remains the same: I am a communicator, catalyst, consciousness raiser, and networker of people and ideas.

Few people even knew I had a brain tumor. When my first symptoms appeared in 1970, I felt as though I had been reborn. I was spiritually a new person, thinking differently, seeing through different eyes. I used to joke, "Taking all those diagnostic tests brainwashed me, washing out a lot of bad stuff from my brain." But somehow it was really true and not a joke. I had a new, better life filled with purpose, meaning, and commitment. I was growing spiritually, with increasing faith in my ability to love and serve others.

The idea for this book originated in 1976 while I was working towards my Master of Arts in Communication degree at Fairfield University in Connecticut. By that time I felt pretty good. While I remained deaf in my left ear, I was no longer an overweight, heavy smoker. I was a normal-weight, non-smoker who exercised daily. And although my left vocal cord remained para-lyzed, I spoke clearly in a new voice.

I enrolled in a class called "Language and Communication." The purpose of the course was "to clarify the role of speech, language, and thought in making humans human." As I looked for a topic for a term paper, a headline on the cover of *Co-Evolution Quarterly* (VOL 16, #2) caught my eye: "Language, Thought and Disease" by W.C. Ellerbroek, MD. On the cover was this quote: "Acne may result from inaccurate self-reporting and be cured by good semantics." Dr. Ellerbroek confirmed what I was already discovering in my own experience: Language is the link between mind, body and emotions. He wrote, "People with acne often feel picked on."

The term "seedthoughts" occurred to me as a convenient summary of the correspondence of language to symptoms. "Seedthoughts" is shorthand for the idea that thoughts affect us physically and emotionally. They can lead to the development of physical symptoms of disease in our bodies . Our thoughts are like seeds that we plant in our minds and hearts. When they germinate they produce wellness or illness.

Gaining Perspective

All these years I'd been my own guinea pig, searching for ways to help myself. I passed on what I learned to others in my role as teacher, counselor, or healer. I used writing and talking to share information. As I talked about these ideas and gave copies of my term paper to people, the ideas expanded.

I had always wanted to write but never knew what to write about. Then, one day, while taking a walk, I realized that I could present my ideas about the language connection and healing in the form of a book. This theme seemed perfect. As soon as I imagined a title in my mind, I recognized that sharing my discoveries and insights was my mission and purpose in life. Little did I know that writing would become part of my healing process.

I wrote the first draft of the first edition in 1983–84. At that time, I assumed that the tumor was gone, or at least removed as a threat to my well-being. For 14 years, I was unaware of any major new symptoms. My voice had become stronger, though talking a lot sometimes tired me. I was still deaf on the left side but it wasn't all bad: I could hear everything I wanted to hear using my right ear. A beneficial side effect was literally being able to turn a deaf ear to unwanted communication. Sleeping on my right side led to total silence.

Writing this book enabled me to know myself better. I recognized that my body expressed my unconscious emotions. For example, I remembered the fears that I began to experience when I first lost my voice and hearing. I wondered which came first, the thought "I lost my nerve" or the loss of the physical nerve energy that resulted from constriction by the tumor. At first I believed that my physical disabilities led to my fearful outlook. My physical condition was — literally and symbolically — an *unnerving* experience.

Today, with the benefit of hindsight, I can see that my physical condition encouraged me to feel the hidden emotions and fears already within me. It enabled me to witness myself being afraid, and with this external dramatization, to realize how fearful I had been for a long time. In other words, the only way I was able to feel my suppressed fears was when they were expressed by way of the nerve damage.

I discovered that by externalizing, verbalizing and examining our hidden emotions in this way, life-threatening illnesses often lead to changes, which in turn allow our emotional and spiritual healing to begin. Personally losing my nerve — feeling fears and developing phobias — showed me what I needed to face in order to heal my spirit. My disabilities led me to the faith I needed to be able to rely on: faith in my abilities; faith in my body and my mind; faith in my relationship to a loving God, where previously I had seen God as a being to be feared. I believe faith coupled with right action may be the best protection any of us has.

Setbacks and Progress

In August, 1984, I read about two Connecticut neurosurgeons who were using lasers to remove brain tumors. I thought their techniques could make surgery on me possible in the unlikely event that my growth was still there. I decided to have a CAT scan to prove once and for all that the tumor was gone. But, I wasn't really as self-confident as I pretended to be. In case the news might be bad, I put off the fearsome CAT scan till November, so that I could finish writing the first draft of my book. At the same time I was acting like the optimist, purposefully leaving space on a page to add the news that the tumor was gone.

In September, 1984, I had my first new symptom in years, in the form of internal pressure which affected my balance. When I stood up after sitting for a long time, I felt a pounding sensation in my head and had difficulty standing straight, until my cerebro-spinal fluid readjusted to my standing up. I was literally being "pressed" to take the diagnostic test.

In November, 1984, the Cat scan proved the tumor had actually grown larger and was pressing on the brain stem. In fact, it had become life-threatening. The doctors said I had less than three years to live unless the tumor was surgically removed.

In February, 1985, I underwent eight hours of brain surgery. The tumor was completely removed. My basic recovery was rapid, with just four days spent in intensive care. But as well as pressing on the brain stem, the tumor had been affecting cranial nerves which transmit neural messages to the body's muscles. I was left disabled, as though I had suffered a stroke. I could hardly talk. Though I was able to think clearly and knew the words to use, my voice was so soft I couldn't be heard. I could barely swallow. I saw double because my eyes didn't focus properly. My face drooped on one side, and the entire left side of my body was weakened. I couldn't walk alone or balance myself. I used a wheelchair for three months.

Fortunately my mind, memory, and intellect remained intact. I managed to keep a journal. My right (writing) hand was okay, and I kept one eye closed in order not to see double. All cranial nerves but the one that governed my tongue remained intact. However, the nerve damage prevented them from working properly. They no longer transmitted the messages which would enable the muscles to fully perform their functions.

My doctors, my family, and I had expected that I would come out of surgery healthy and able to resume my life as before. Instead, I spent three weeks in Bridgeport Hospital and four weeks at Gaylord, a wonderful Connecticut rehabilitation center.

After coming home my progress speeded up. I soon looked great. Function returned quickly to my facial muscles and I learned ways to eat almost everything, even with the swallowing problems. My eyes improved after three months. I could read and watch television. More importantly, I could work. I began writing again, eventually completely revising the first pre-surgery draft of this book.

Everything improved, slowly or rapidly, depending on whose perspective was involved. For a time I walked a bit like a wobbling toddler or a staggering drunk. I still carry a cane when I walk in the woods or during snowy, icy weather. Typing is somewhat difficult because my left side is not well-coordinated.

In 1987 I had another operation, this time at Yale Medical Center which strengthened my voice by allowing my right working vocal cord to vibrate off the paralyzed left one. Within a year, I could drive, supporting my desire for independence. With each healing milestone, I thanked God and told myself *"Somebody up there loves me."*

New Perspective

It has not all been bad. During that first year after surgery I was given the gift of time for those things I had often wanted to do but neglected — like reading the Bible. I found biblical roots for much of what I believed and wrote about. That amazed me.

I was encouraged by the faith of Christian evangelists on TV. Their messages gave me hope for healing. I took time to listen to different spiritual teachers on cassette tapes and meditate on their words. I saw anew how I had been guided by a Higher Power all along. I prayed and talked to God many hours each day. I rediscovered my Jewish roots and with them a renewed desire to love and serve humanity. Eventually, I returned to Judaism and found a missing part of myself and a healthier, more satisfying, way of life.

There were moments of great happiness. My husband, my sister, and my children stood by me. Realizing the depth of their love was a great gift. The love and care I received from family, friends, and even strangers was incredible. Many people prayed for me, and I felt their love in the darkest times. One dear friend prayed and fasted for me the day of my surgery. Before the surgery, I called some telephone prayer services and asked for prayers, something I still do at times. With my family and my personal relationship with God, I felt safe and protected, believing I would make it through.

Though I had periods of feeling sorry for myself, I also saw how blessed I was by what I could do easily, like tying my shoes. Gaylord Rehabilitation Center was filled with people who were worse off than me. I was in tough straits, but at least my prognosis was hopeful. As the old adage goes, "I felt sorry for myself because I had no shoes — and then I met a man who had no feet." The end result of the whole process is that I am tougher now, more at peace and faith-filled. Compared to the hell I was in right after surgery, I'm in heaven now.

I have found that personal growth is always a challenge. My circumstances gave me the opportunity to overcome frustration and release fear, exercise faith, learn trust and patience, and surrender control to a wise and loving Higher Power. Progress seemed so slight at first. I kept remembering words of wisdom told me by my husband ages ago, "The strength of your growth will be your belief without proof." Faith is indeed belief without proof. During the times when life didn't seem worth living, I was strengthened by that seed of faith planted within me. Though I now have strong faith, I still look for proof. And proof comes in bits and pieces, with each subtle change in me. But the faith came first.

Throughout my healing I used the tools that I describe in this book. For example, visualization: Each time a therapist taught me some new maneuver, like how to stand up, I practiced it in my mind as well as with my body. As a result my physical therapy went smoothly and I gained strength and ability quickly.

The healing of my nervous system will continue for years and my prognosis remains excellent. However, in the natural or physical world, no health care professional will guarantee how much healing will occur. But in the spiritual world, God's word promises me healing. Since we tend to get what we believe, I still live on those words, believing in my eventual full recovery. I believe in The Spiritual Law of Agreement: our shared belief, focused on a goal, activates a tremendous amount of healing power. Some people call that the power of prayer.

Getting sick, paralyzed, deaf, and afraid enabled me to write this book from a point of deep personal understanding. I am now allowing my healing and release from fear to joy, from disability to enabledness, from imperfection to perfection, from burden to unconditional love and service. I thank God and my doctors for saving me from the tumor, allowing this great adventure to continue. It really was a miracle. I acknowledge myself as well for my willingness to undertake this project and see it through to completion. This book — about the kinds of thoughts, images, and words which can help us to heal — is part of my thanks.

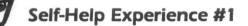

Self-Help Experience #1

Practice in Self-Awareness Makes Perfect

Purpose: This exercise will add to your self-knowledge by helping you to recognize your emotions and their effect on you physically. Read through all the instructions first and then follow them with your eyes closed. Have a pen and paper ready to make notes after the exercise. Find a quiet place where you will not be disturbed for a few minutes. Relax and then begin.

Can you recall a time when you realized you were really unhappy about a situation? Perhaps you didn't want to face that unhappiness. Perhaps you thought that admitting you were angry, hurt, or sad would lead you into trouble, letting you feel or do something that you didn't want to feel or do. When you recognize and release those emotions, your body becomes healthier and more relaxed.

When you are ill, you are guided into right action by observing your symptoms as metaphors—symbols that may represent the root cause. Be prepared for those times by practicing observing what you are experiencing right now. Don't judge— just observe yourself. In other words, at least during this exercise, accept your feelings. Don't put yourself down for what you are feeling.

Use this technique of *witnessing yourself* when you feel physical or emotional pain, or tension. You can put the following instructions on a tape recorder to play back to yourself or have a friend read them to you. Be sure to pause, leaving some quiet time after reading or recording each instruction.

Instructions

1. Take a comfortable position either sitting or lying down. Relax.

2. Allow your attention to rest or focus on different parts of your body — from your toes to the top of your head.

3. Describe to yourself what you are feeling physically and emotionally at this very moment.

4. Notice the thoughts you are thinking.

5. Recall an unhappy incident and repeat steps 2-4. Notice if there is a change in your thoughts, feelings or emotions from the way you felt before recalling the unhappy incident. Pause for a few minutes.

6. Stop thinking about the unhappy memory. Release it completely. Now recall a different situation, one that made you angry. Repeat steps 2-4. Become aware of any change in your thoughts, feelings or emotions. Pause for a few moments.

7. Stop thinking about the angry memory. Release it completely. Finally recall a happy time and repeat the first 4 steps. Again notice any change in your thoughts, feelings and emotions. Pause.

8. Smile to yourself.

9. Open your eyes and review what you've learned about yourself, your emotions and your body during this self-witnessing experience. It can help if you write down what you've learned though this is not necessary to the success of the exercise.

Every so often during the day, check your body for tension. For example, check your hands. Are they clenched or open? How about your mouth—are you gritting your teeth? Are you smiling? Frequent daily body checks will enhance self-awareness. Practice does make perfect—perfect self-awareness.

A primary benefit of this exercise is that you will be more aware of your own feelings and empowered to identify your typical responses to those feelings. This awareness gives you the freedom to choose your future actions, rather than the automatic knee-jerk reactions typical of many people. You can learn to choose how you will respond to your emotions when you are aware of their effects on you.

Happiness is a butterfly which, when pursued,
is always beyond our grasp, but, if you will sit
down quietly, may alight upon you.
—Nathaniel Hawthorne

Which came first, the chicken or the egg?

He pined away and died of grief.

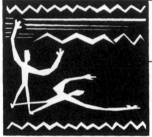

Chapter 2

The Fundamentals of Healing

Long ago, people recognized the interconnectedness of mind, body, and spirit and its relationship to health. For centuries it was taken for granted that people could "die of grief," that unrequited love could cause a person to "pine away," that fear could make one "deathly afraid," that anger could cause illness.

Then, in the nineteenth century, the germ theory of disease implicated bacteria in infections, which had been responsible for much illness and death throughout the centuries. Unfortunately, the discovery of the role of germs in causing disease impeded the previous understanding of the link between emotions and health.

Today medicine is adept at eliminating the effects of bacteria and some viruses through improved sanitation, vaccination and powerful drugs. Yet drugs do not heal or regrow damaged tissue. Furthermore, suppression of symptoms at times leads to problems of cell degeneration — problems often more serious than the original infection.

Even so, many mainstream medical practitioners (with the exception of psychiatrists) continue to ignore the role of the mind and emotions in causing and healing disease. Conventional, so-called allopathic medicine focuses on unwanted physical sensations or symptoms and their suppression or alteration. Mainstream doctors use drugs and surgery to suppress or remove symptoms. Alternative health care professionals such as Naturopaths, Homeopaths and Chiropractors might use food, herbs or bodily manipulations to relieve symptoms. Yet in many cases different symptoms replace the original ones. Removing a symptom doesn't necessarily lead to healing or a cure.

Why do some people suffer illnesses when exposed to viruses and bacteria while others, exposed to the same microorganisms, remain healthy? Even with the idea that fatigue, weakness, and prior illnesses lower one's resistance to infection, the germ theory provides only a partial explanation of illness. Traditionally, each symptom or set of symptoms is considered a separate disease entity, ignoring the emotional connections linking the new set of symptoms to a previous disease.

Holistic Medicine

Today, holistic medicine helps heal the patient by providing a whole viewpoint. It views the patient from the total perspective of body, mind, and spirit. Each of these is an aspect of being human and no part can be eliminated if full healing is to occur. Holistic medical practice includes orthodox medical approaches to each of these human aspects, as well as alternative therapies. It represents the cooperation of traditional and non-traditional approaches. This is what Dr. Robert Atkins calls "complementary medicine" in his book *Dr. Atkins' Health Revolution*. Increasingly, mainstream medical doctors are adopting some of these non-traditional approaches, particularly those that have been subjected to scientific examination.

Holistic medicine doesn't ignore bacteria, viruses, or any physical causes of disease. Rather, this approach recognizes many causal factors, including some traditional ones like heredity and environment. These causal factors are integrated with the knowledge of the power of the mind and emotions to predispose us to health or illness.

Holistic medicine increasingly understands the role language plays in translating thoughts and emotions into physical conditions. The mind's power lies in its ability to think, reason, remember, and create images. With our conscious awareness, we choose the images and thoughts we want to focus on. Some images support well-being while others encourage the illness and suffering that continue to ravage humanity. Today many more doctors accept the idea that emotions affect the body even if they don't understand how or why.

A good doctor knows that what you tell yourself about what happens to you makes a very deep impression. How you feel about your current and past life circumstances, including what you tell yourself about them, can add stress to your life, or make the stress less damaging. Holistic healing professionals take time to talk to their patients, to really listen to their ideas, to explore the emotional component of any symptoms the patient is experiencing. A truly holistic doctor understands that talking things out helps to prevent and/or relieve the physical symptoms related to an emotional experience.

Dr. Marvin Schweitzer, a member of my personal team of health helpers, is a Naturopathic Doctor or N.D. practicing in Norwalk, Connecticut. A Naturopath has years of training similar to a Medical Doctor, but instead of learning about and using drugs, Naturopaths learn more about natural things like food and herbs—nature's botanical medicines. Schweitzer's practice is structured in a way that allows him time to really get to know his patients.

Schweitzer told me, "I can't understand why everyone doesn't practice this way. It's so rewarding. A person's quality of life does not depend solely on his current health status but also on their attitude towards the illness—towards whatever is going on. Two people can have the identical diagnosis, yet one person's life is a living hell, while the other person's life is filled with happiness. When a person is living fully and with joy — no matter what the circumstances — that opens my heart. That person inspires me and becomes my teacher."[1]

Currently, more medical doctors are adopting a similar philosophy. Another member of my health care team is Dr. Robban Sica, a medical doctor in Orange, Connecticut, who takes a holistic approach to treating and preventing illness. In describing her way of practicing medicine, she said:

"I strive to integrate the best of conventional medicine (such as standard diagnostic techniques, blood work, and medications when necessary) with the best of alternative medicine. Taking time to listen to the patient is essential. A wise teacher of mine once said that at least 50% of the healing process is being fully present and listening. Even if we can't make the symptoms go away, people feel better for having been heard.

"In my experience, most people want and need to be empowered to take charge of their health. Part of my job is to help them to sort out which factors are affecting them and to choose from a broad range of holistic healing techniques.

"I like to keep in mind the medical credo of 'first do no harm.' Therefore, I feel comfortable using harmless techniques such as meditation, daily exercise, biofeedback, or nutritional changes that help people feel better, while we are waiting for the scientific evidence. While it's satisfying and comforting to have studies documenting these effects, it would also be a shame to make patients wait in order to benefit."[2]

Ridding the Body of Disease-Causing Pollutants

Pollution can be seen as a common factor in most illnesses—pollution of the body with toxic wastes and pollution of the mind with negative thoughts. Both may lead to emotions like depression, anger, resentment, and so on. Digestive pollution comes from eating the wrong foods or overeating in general. Environmental pollution puts stress on the physical body and reduces its resistance. Language pollution comes from using negative words and dwelling on fearful thoughts that create harmful stress. All three pollutions are usually present in disease. Everything that isn't in harmony with the body pollutes it. We get well by releasing our pollution.

If you give a body a chance, it has the means to destroy illness-causing agents. We cleanse ourselves of most digestive and environmental pollutants through rest, fasting, dietary choices and fever. For example, the heat of a fever activates the antibodies in the blood and lymph system to stop germs. Symptoms like fever, swelling, and discharge may be the very means the body uses to heal itself, by releasing some of the pollutants. Even crying and deep breathing can release pollutants. Suppressing these symptoms may interfere with the deeper healing process.

On the other hand, listening to the message of one's disease and then taking appropriate action gives the body a chance to heal itself by using its own defensive systems.

After ridding the body of infectious or toxic material, the next step is to alter the underlying thought patterns and emotional stresses that allow germs to take root. Mental and emotional fasting — thinking thoughts that won't invite germs in — helps the body to remain free of illness and disease. This kind of self-healing often strengthens the body's future resistance to disease.

At the present time we are adept at removing the symptoms of illness using medicines and surgery, but few people know how to use the mind as a tool for healing the physical body. The average person can't even conceive that he might cause himself illness or that he can "uncause" that illness by changing destructive thought patterns and altering self-damaging behaviors. These are not skills we are generally taught. Yet using them we can release the mind's language pollution.

Many people feel more comfortable in the role of victim of disease. They want a doctor to do something to make them better. The idea of taking a drug to cure a disease seems simpler to accept than the idea of self-healing. And it may be easier for most people. But as researchers recognize the increasingly toxic side effects of many drugs, it is prudent to seek other less intrusive, more natural, and often less costly healing techniques.

A doctor's responsibility is to use his training to help you to help yourself. But final responsibility for your health rests with you. You decide whether to use what's available or not.

Psychosomatics

At the turn of the century, Sir William Osler — a medical giant — anticipated psychosomatic medicine by declaring, "The care of tuberculosis depends more on what the patient has in his head than what he has in his chest."

Psychosomatic (both physiological and psychological) medicine does recognize the role of mind and emotions in disease. But when psychosomatic medicine was first popularized, many people perceived the label "psychosomatic illness" as derogatory. "Psychosomatic" came to mean "all in the mind" or unreal. It became jargon for "hypochondriac." It implied that the patient was not really feeling the symptoms but only making them up. Some people even thought they were crazy when told that what they felt was not real. To many people, any reference to "mind" in an illness meant "crazy." "It's all in your mind" was a diagnosis to be feared.

The reality of the matter is that disease is often a *product* of the mind, and not "all in the mind." The mental and emotional causes of disease produce real physical effects. When you are feeling ill, you are actually feeling ill no matter what the cause.

Old-fashioned psychosomatic medicine often seemed to imply that some illnesses were real and others were not. "Real" illness implied physical or organic change or damage. Thus, "not real" illness — meaning non-physical — was all in your mind. Holistic medicine is rapidly changing that idea by recognizing that you do actually feel within your body sensations that result from an event in your mind.

Sometimes your body reacts and you may not be aware of any physical sensations. Hypertension (high blood pressure) often reflects this truth. You have a physical reaction to emotional pressures. You may learn about your bodily reaction only after having a blood pressure reading.

Any emotion from laughter to sadness to fear provokes a physiological response. There is no such thing as all in your mind. There is the mental component of your feelings and the physical reaction of your body.

Contemporary Mind-Body Perspectives

Joan Borysenko has a Ph.D. in cellular biology from Harvard Medical School. She co-founded the Mind/Body Clinic at Beth Israel Hospital in Boston. Dr. Borysenko's main research interest is the effect of mind on immunity. In her book *Minding the Body, Mending the Mind*, writing about neuropeptides (hormonal messengers) she says, "there is a rich and intricate two-way communication system linking the mind, the immune system, and potentially all other systems, a pathway through which our emotions — our hopes and fears — can affect the body's ability to defend itself.[3]

"In laboratory experiments, we've learned that stress, whether acute or chronic, releases a whole array of hormones that provide quick energy. Two of these hormones — adrenaline and cortisol—are also potent inhibitors of the immune system."[4]

In one study[5] that Dr. Borysenko conducted with her husband, immunologist Dr. Myrin Borysenko, Dr. Bruce Crary, and Dr. Herbert Benson, volunteers were injected with a tiny dose of adrenaline — enough to produce the same reaction in you if someone yelled, "Boo." Blood tests revealed an immediate decline in lymphocytes, the helper cells that augment the response of the immune system. This shows the immediate effect that fear has on the body at a cellular level.

In another study, this one using dental students, Borysenko, her husband, and other colleagues discovered "that the stress of examination periods reduced the level of a particular antibody in saliva, an antibody that is part of the first line of defense against colds. Exam time is typically when students are most likely to catch colds."[6] After psychological testing of their subjects, they further concluded that students with a more easygoing attitude showed less of a drop in antibodies than the other students. Borysenko noted studies by doctors at Ohio State confirm that exam stress reduces the effectiveness of lymphocyte cells whose function is the destruction of virus-infected and cancerous cells.

Borysenko writes, "Disease, however, is rarely a simple matter of isolated cause and effect. While stress and helplessness can depress immune function, clearly we don't get sick each time we're stressed. It's far more reasonable to consider stress as one of many factors that may tip the balance toward illness."[7]

The brain-mind connection in disease as evidenced in the mouth has been well-known and well-documented for many years. Connecticut periodontist, Dr. Randall Neichen, D.D.S., learned about the mind-body connection in gum disease years ago while in dental school. He said "During World War Two, Acute Necrotizing Ulcerative Gingivitis [ANUG], a disease commonly known as *Trench Mouth* was thought to be contagious as it was universally present in the mouths of soldiers in the trenches. Notwithstanding the fact that under such conditions these young man weren't able to brush, they were all under the same stress. One can imagine the fear present in the minds of young men living in trenches, battling the all too real enemies of World War II. After the war it was recognized that Trench Mouth wasn't contagious after all but a stress related disorder. During exam time college students often suffer the same problem with ANUG."[8]

Norman Cousins, well-known editor and author of *Anatomy of an Illness* among other books, wrote about how he used laughter to help cure a stress-produced "incurable" collagen disease. By laughing heartily at movies of his favorite comedians, he was able to get pain-free, drug-free sleep and a boost toward full recovery. Science has since learned that love, laughter ("internal jogging" as Cousins calls it), and other positive emotions and actions rally the body's natural defenses against stress, pain, and disease. Laughing at jokes, at the human condition, and at yourself can help you live longer and happier.

Recognizing that the will to live, the capacity for joy, and self-confidence are important components of total health care, not alternatives to orthodox medicine, Cousins wrote, "The wise physician favors a spirit of responsible participation by the patients in a total strategy of medical care...There has been enough replication of research involving controlled studies to point to a presiding fact; namely the physician has a prime resource at his disposal in the form of the patient's own apothecary, especially when combined with the prescription pad."[9]

Your thoughts, fears, and emotions often stimulate detectable physical conditions, though you are almost never conscious of this link or in conscious control of it. But the implications of this discovery are stunning: *if you make disease happen, you also have the power to change it, even to get rid of it.* Disease often forces people to alter negative thoughts, useless behaviors, and ill feelings.

From the poly-pharmacy of more than fifty hormones produced in your brain which stimulate the various organs of your body, your mind does influence matter. The reverse is also true: your *mind* is influenced by *matter.* Through the power of your mind, you control the matter that is your body and vice versa. Anything that interferes with the production and dispersal of these hormones has an impact on your body, your mind and your emotions.

Sometimes the hormonal connection between body and mind is influenced by outside sources, such as sunlight. This provides a medical explanation for the depressions and lethargy suffered by millions of people living in northern areas during the fall and winter months. Scientists have labelled this condition as SAD, for Seasonal Affective Disorder.

Research has shown that lack of sunlight affects brain chemistry, which in turn affects mood. Fortunately the use of special full spectrum lights for up to 30 minutes per day bring back health and well being in up to 80 percent of people with SAD symptoms. According to Dr. Martin Teicher, chief of the chronobiology laboratory at McLean Hospital in Belmont, Massachusetts, "People who talked of hating winter all of a sudden become fans of winter."[10] When the body works properly and one feels physically better, then more positive thoughts and attitudes follow.

Emotion's Effect on the Body

A recent hour spent electronically "surfing the Internet" turned up reports of research on the many ways emotions affect our bodies. The Institute of HeartMath[11] presented numerous studies which show that emotions can affect a variety of physiological systems, including cardiovascular, nervous, immune and hormonal systems. They demonstrate the effects of stress and mental and emotional states on the electrophysiology of the body.

For example, anger and appreciation each can affect the balance of the autonomic nervous system. In one Institute research study, it was shown that negative emotions such as anger, or positive emotions such as appreciation, have a direct effect on heart rate variability.[12] In another study, subjects were able to double their level of DHEA, an anti-aging hormone, and reduce their level of cortisol, a stress hormone, by 23 percent in just one month of regularly practicing techniques taught at HeartMath Institute.[13]

Stress and depression send hormones flowing into the blood stream, making people more susceptible to disease, particularly cancer. Journalist Andy Geller[14] reported in a *New York Post* article headlined *You Can Worry Yourself Sick Over Latest Cancer Study*: "The 'fight or flight' reflex that once gave humans the speed and endurance to escape primitive dangers is triggered daily in modern people, keeping their hormones in a state of constant hyper-readiness, researchers said yesterday."

Experts also said that "people with weak immune systems caused by high stress-hormone levels also are more likely to become infected with viruses linked to cancer."

Geller cited a study by Dr. Janice Kiecolt-Glaser which showed that routine marital disagreements can cause the "fight or flight" reaction "which floods the bloodstream with hormones which can ultimately cause damage to the body."[15] Kiecolt-Glaser took frequent blood samples during interviews with newlywed couples. When the interview led to disagreement or argument, women proved exceptionally sensitive and released higher levels of stress hormones. So women ultimately might suffer long term from the increased hormonal levels during a marital spat. And there thus might be some truth to the anecdotally reported notion of some holistic healers that anger toward men is a factor in breast cancer.

Journalist Geller then quoted Dr. Philip Gold of The National Institute of Mental Health who spoke on the effects of stress and depression on physical disease: "Some forms of depression bring on a similar hormonal state. In many people these hormones turn on and stay on for a long time."[16] High levels of the emergency hormones also cause brittle bones in women. Gold presented a study of bone density in forty-year-old women. Those who were depressed had high levels of stress hormones and the bone density of 70 year olds, making them much more susceptible to fractures. Such studies confirm that emotions trigger a body response which can ultimately lead to long range damage.

Body and Mind: Functionally Inseparable

Just as nose and thumb refer to different parts of one body, *mind* and *body* refer to different aspects of the same whole. Every emotion you feel and every thought you think is also a physical event. Though mind and body are inseparable, dictionaries often define words such as "mind" and "body," "mental" and "physical," and "psychic" and "somatic" as antonyms or opposites. Actually they are *functionally* inseparable. Both aspects of self must be present for a human to be a fully alive human. I'll not address the idea of soul or spirit at this time except to say that I believe that there is something beyond my body/mind (a consciousness greater than my individual self.)

Dr. David Graham of the University of Wisconsin Medical School calls mind-versus-body terminology *linguistic dualism.* "The convenience of the separation exists, but it is important to remember that this is nothing more than a linguistic convenience. It is in direct opposition to the way you actually work."[17] Just as the water and the land overlap at the shore, the body and mind have many points of intersection. Rivers and streams flow above and below ground until they finally merge and find full expression in the sea. So too, emotions and thoughts often express themselves in the physical body.

"Psychological" and "physical" and their synonyms refer to *different ways of talking about the same event.* Acne, for example, has a physical component — reddening of the skin, eruptions on the face, chest or back containing toxic material and often painful sensations. Acne has a psychological component as well: it can *cause* depression or *result from* depression. People with this condition often think they look ugly and fear others will reject them. Depending on the severity of the condition, emotions such as shame or embarrassment may result.

Others with acne may react in a very different way. They may believe acne is an inevitable result of adolescence that will pass. Still others may not mind their condition, believing acne is a way for the body to rid itself of wastes through the skin. The event "acne" is a multi-dimensional experience. Thus there are different perspectives from which to view a disease process, including physical and psychological.

The medical profession has encouraged the mind/body division by often ignoring the mind when treating physical symptoms. It unnaturally divided the body into parts and organs, implicitly undermining the reality that every part of the body, every organ, affects every other. The medical profession in general, and medical specialists in their fields, have brought us enormous benefits, and their contribution should not be downplayed. But specialists have sometimes been limited because they saw their patients as series of parts to be healed rather than as whole human beings. By forgetting about the body's mental and emotional connections, we may not recognize the creative role of the mind in all physical disease. Though words and thoughts alone don't cause disease, thoughts affect us by triggering responses in the body which lead to chemical, hormonal, neurological, and muscular changes.

When we began to define the parts of the body by their functions — the heart is just a pump, the stomach is a sack, hearing is the result of some bones vibrating in the head, muscles are pulleys — we moved away from understanding man as greater than the sum of his parts, and ceased understanding the wholeness of man at all. It's important to understand how each part works, but something valuable often gets lost in the process. Ronald J. Glasser, M.D., in *The Body Is The Hero* wrote, "we know, even if our surgeons and internists don't, that we are connected with our bodies, that the catch in our breath when we are startled, the tension in our guts when we're worried, the exhaustion we feel from our anxiety are as much a part of our illnesses as are the bacteria, viruses and auto-antibodies which attack us, and can in fact be just as debilitating and just as deadly."[18] To fully cure anyone of anything, it's important to treat the whole patient, mind and emotions as well as body.

Some cultures continue to recognize that all parts of the human are involved in the disease process. Medicine men and shamans treat both mind and body. Through potions and incantations they work on the physical and spiritual levels. The use of these rituals releases negativity and opens one's mind to believing that healing will occur. Medicine men and some present-day western healers recognize that a mind open to the possibility of healing encourages the process to begin and move more easily to completion.

Thought Affects Physiology

Physicist and psychologist Buryl Payne, Ph.D., writes:

"We know that thoughts generated in the brain activate hormone secretions and stimulate other nerve centers within the body. Thoughts, coded as neural impulses, travel along nerve axons, activating muscles and glands similar to the manner in which telephone messages travel over wires in the form of electrical signals. Experiments with the GSR, a biofeedback instrument, attached to fingers or toes clearly demonstrate that mental activity reaches into the extremities of the body.

"With sensitive EMG instruments, we can show that muscles are activated when we think about anything involving action or emotion, even though there may be no visible movement. Although we do not know how thoughts are generated in the brain, it seems clear that once present, thoughts are amplified by the brain and turned into actions. Every thought we think influences millions of atoms, molecules, and cells throughout the body. Besides this straightforward effect on the physical body, we know from general principles of physics that any acceleration of electrons produces some electromagnetic radiation."[19]

Biofeedback instruments demonstrate the effect of thoughts and emotions on the body, for instance by proving that muscles are activated when we think about anything involving action. According to writer Bette Runck, "Biofeedback is a treatment technique in which people are trained to improve their health by using signals from their own bodies. Physical therapists use biofeedback to help stroke victims regain movement in paralyzed muscles. Psychologists use it to help tense and anxious clients learn to relax. Specialists in many different fields use biofeedback to help their patients cope with pain."[20]

Among the many biofeedback tools that can help us recognize how our body is behaving are *thermometers*, which measure body temperature; *sphygmomanometers*, which measure blood pressure; and *electromyography (EMG)*, which measures electric currents associated with muscular action and hence body relaxation. A beeper on the EMG alerts the subject when certain muscles become too tense. Used in re-training body responses, the EMG is a powerful tool for releasing stress and increasing self-knowledge.

Until I experienced biofeedback I never realized how tense I had been when having my blood pressure taken. Trying to relax, I often became more tense. I would shut my eyes and hold my breath, leading to increased body tension. This is obvious to me now, but I was less conscious at the time, and thought I was relaxing. To train me, a psychologist guided me through Progressive Muscle Relaxation (a technique explained in self-help experience #2 at the end of this chapter.) When I was successful in turning off the beeper, the EMG confirmed objectively the depth of relaxation I subjectively felt.

There is ample documentation in the medical literature of the effects of strong emotion on the human body. Strong emotions are triggered by moving events or experiences. Emotions are real, primal, instinctive—raw feelings triggered by events and experiences and sometimes by the experience of a thought. But usually thoughts are our attempt to give meaning to our emotions. The quality of our thoughts determines how well we cope with emotional experiences and influences whether we feel well or dis-eased. People can literally die after being "scared to death."

Norman Cousins cites a study, reported by George Engel, of people who died in response to shattering news. In the study 27 percent of the people who died suddenly from emotional shock had been confronted with "grave" personal danger. Engel in turn quoted another study by J.C. Barker, which described forty-two cases of people who died abruptly after being frightened. Cousins comments, "Folklore and medical science come together in accepting the reality of sudden death through emotional causes. Folklore makes note of the fact; medical science understands what happens inside the body to bring it about."[21] Apparently sudden emotional shock may touch off a dangerously rapid and erratic heartbeat, technically known as fibrillation. Cousins's theme is that "nothing is more essential in the treatment of serious disease than liberating the patient from panic and foreboding."[22]

Grief, too, is a potent emotional force. A person can literally "die of a broken heart." James J. Lynch, Scientific Director of the Psychosomatic Clinics at the University of Maryland School of Medicine has this to say about the effects of human companionship on health: "the 'broken heart' is not just a poetic image for loneliness and despair—it is a medical reality. In our fragmented society, the lack of human companionship—chronic loneliness and social isolation as well as the sudden loss of loved ones—is one of the leading causes of premature death. And while lack of human companionship is related to virtually every major disease from cancer and tuberculosis to mental illness, the link is particularly marked in the case of heart disease, the nation's leading killer. Every year millions die, quite literally, of a broken or lonely heart."[23]

Strong emotions can produce the physiological changes that allow disease conditions to flourish. These strong emotions are often triggered by thoughts. Dr. Andrew Weil M.D.[24] is an authoritative and important voice on the subject of health and healing today. He wrote about the healing system within the body which is responsible, not only for remissions of life-threatening diseases but also, for day-to-day maintenance and for positive responses to everyday illnesses. Speaking on "The Phil Donohue Show" as far back as June of 1987 he said, "Disordered thinking can produce disordered brain chemistry."

Orderly thinking can produce orderly brain chemistry. By noticing such harmful thoughts as "I am sick and tired of that," or "she drives me crazy," or "he makes me sick," or even "I am scared to death" you will begin to recognize your own connections between language and disease. With this increased awareness you can begin to eliminate those thoughts and feel for yourself if there is a change in your level of well-being.

Harnessing the Positive Power of Attitudes

My son Steven, a CPA, offers good advice: "You have to learn not to absorb pressure from negative situations. You absorb pressure when people or situations make unreasonable demands on you and you let that get the best of you. It's better to exert your own pressure to transform the demand and improve the situation rather than take it into yourself and make yourself ill."[25] In other words, *take whatever is happening and make use of it.*

For example, those with cancer often begin using techniques such as visualization and meditation which reportedly help to strengthen their immune systems thus improving their chances of survival. They often *feel* better just by actively participating in their healing process. Furthermore, many of these cancer victims start seeing themselves as survivors who have benefited from their bout with cancer. Serious illness often encourages us to look at what is really important to us.

"When faced with a life threatening illness or other crisis, people often make dramatic changes they never thought possible. A New Zealand research team questioned heart attack and cancer patients about positive changes in their lives following their illness. 51% reported healthy lifestyle changes. 28% reported a greater appreciation of life and health. 24% reported improved close relationships. Other common changes included a shift in personal priorities, greater knowledge of health, feeling fortunate to be given a second chance and improved empathy towards others."[26]

Changing one's thoughts and improving one's attitude can enhance immune function leading to near miraculous results. Paul Pearsall, Ph.D., in his book *Superimmunity* reports on the results of Drs. Elmer and Alyce Green's examination of four hundred cases of spontaneous remissions in cancer patients. He defines spontaneous remission as "all of a sudden the disease went away and we have no idea why, and we didn't seem to do anything to make it go away based on our treatment." The Greens "found only one factor common to each case they examined. All these people had changed their attitude prior to the remission and, in some way, had found hope and become more positive in their approach to the disease."[27]

Pearsall writes, "It puzzles me that physicians sometimes forget that the bombardment of the system with deadly chemicals against cancer is also related to how we feel and that spontaneous remissions occur during these treatment regimens as well. Studies on the successes of radiation and chemotherapy seldom report on changes in the belief systems and attitudes of the patients receiving the treatment. It seems equally plausible that people's belief systems change when an encouraging, trusted doctor, in this case serving in the role of shaman or healer, administers a magic elixir in the form of strong chemicals or buzzing machines that alter not only cell biology but personal psychology."[28] A very useful, well-documented, book on this subject of who gets well and why is *Remarkable Recovery: What Extraordinary Healings Tell Us About Getting Well And Staying Well* by Caryle Hirshberg and Marc Barasch.

We have come full circle as research proves that your mind, your body and your emotions are linked in a sometimes delicate balance. Upset the balance in one area and disease can result in any other area—sometimes just leading to emotional unhappiness and sometimes leading to acute or chronic physical damage. Maintaining a proper balance essential for good health and a sense of well-being often begins with the recognition of the interconnectedness of your mental, physical and emotional sides. The holistic path to healing including nutritional, spiritual, and psychological approaches along with medical protocols and technology seems the wisest course for any seriously ill patient. Perhaps the cure for all disease is rooted in the holistic concept that *to cure someone of an illness, one must not only release a specific symptom but deal with underlying and corollary causes.*

As information about the power of words and thoughts becomes even more widespread, the role of mind in healing is subject to increasing research. The search for medicines that assist in healing will continue. And since numerous research studies in the field of psychoneuroimmunology suggest that people can voluntarily enhance their immune systems,[29] the search for newer, more powerful mental technology should also continue. Someday even conventional researchers may find the cure for cancer, AIDS and other serious illnesses by focusing on patients' beliefs, attitudes and willingness to change as well as new treatments and more potent drugs.

Self-Help Experience #2
Progressive Muscle Relaxation

Purpose: To help you to be more in touch with the feel of different parts of your body and to assist you in relaxing your body.

During biofeedback training I realized that I didn't know how to tense certain parts of my body, because I often couldn't differentiate a tense muscle from a relaxed one. My tense muscles weren't initially responsive to my conscious control. Chronically tense or contracted muscles reveal a habitual response pattern in one's life—usually below one's conscious level of awareness. Practice in tensing and releasing ultimately leads to increased awareness and a finely-tuned ability to release tension more easily.

Progressive muscle relaxation is an exercise to de-stress and relax your body. It involves clenching and releasing muscles in different parts of the body. Your eyes may be open or shut, though focusing within is easier with eyes shut.

Instructions:

1. Begin by getting into a relaxed position, either lying down or sitting in a comfortable chair.

2. Clench your right hand into a fist.

3. Observe the sensations in your hand, arm, shoulder, and elsewhere in your body, for a few seconds.

4. Release your fist by opening your hand and relaxing it.

5. Notice the differences in sensation between the clenched and the released state.

6. Do this process several times.

7. Tighten your stomach muscles. Observe your physical sensations in your stomach and in the rest of your body.

8. Relax your stomach muscles and notice how you feel. Tighten and relax a few times.

9. Contract your buttocks. Notice how this feels. Then release the tightened buttocks muscles and observe how you feel.

10. Contract the muscles of your head and face including your eyes, your forehead, your cheeks, and chin. How does each one feel? Relax the muscles and observe the differences in feeling.

As you become adept at this clenching and releasing process, you can isolate any part of your body you wish to work on. Pay special attention to the head, neck, shoulders, lower back and stomach. It takes about twenty minutes per session until you master the process. At the end of each practice session, stop actively tensing. Then, just *imagine* your fist being clenched. Don't do it. Just *think* it. Notice if you are still relaxed. After several weeks of performing this process, you will feel less tense. You may discover *where* in your body you are holding tension. In places where you are chronically tense, you may not be aware of the muscles until you begin to release the tension.

> *Drag your thoughts away from your troubles —by the*
> *ears, by the heels, or any other way you can manage it.*
> *It's the healthiest thing a body can do.*
> *—Mark Twain*

Self-Help Experience #3

The Pendulum

Purpose: To observe the energy of a thought affecting your body.

You can test the effects of your thoughts on your body by trying the following experiment. Use a necklace with a pendant, or tie a weight (like a ring) on a piece of string, in order to create a pendulum. Sit in a relaxed position, with the elbow of the arm that is holding the pendulum resting on a table. Think about the pendulum moving, but don't make it move by

(continued, next page)

moving your arm. Tell yourself that you *will* the pendulum to move. You may suggest the direction (sideways, front–to–back, or diagonally) or not. Holding the pendulum without trying to move it in any way, allow the pendulum to move by itself.

You can keep your eyes closed until you seem to feel the pendulum moving—then you can peek. You will be amazed how your thoughts cause the pendulum to swing without you moving your hand. Some minute neuromuscular mechanism controlled subconsciously is probably at work, something so subtle that most of us are not aware of it.

Let us train our minds to desire what the situation demands.
—*Seneca*

Self-Help Experience #4

Harmonizing Your Thoughts

Purpose: To determine how and to what degree your thoughts affect you emotionally and physically. This exercise provides practice in observing and releasing unwanted thoughts and letting go of obsessions.

Notice what types of thoughts improve your sense of well-being and what circumstances surround those thoughts. The average person has thousands of thoughts a day—some we call *positive*: hopes, dreams, memories of happy times, loving feelings, and so on; some we call *negative*: worries, jealousies, insecurities, angers, cravings for forbidden things.

Some people believe we need to accept negative thoughts. In a sense that's true. We can learn much about ourselves from our so-called negative thoughts. But we must also be able to let them go. Identifications of thought as "positive" and "negative" are based on our own mental judgments.

Sometimes we get stuck in thinking about an experience. We

dwell on it so much that we can't get on with life. To restore harmony within, you must learn to "get off it," to change the place where your mind is dwelling. *You can choose what to think,* which will influence how you feel. If an unwanted thought spontaneously arises, you can rid yourself of that thought by replacing it with another thought of your choice. *The mind can only think one complete thought at a time.* After a while it will become second nature for you to replace your unwanted negative thoughts with desirable positive ones.

Instructions

1. For the next few days, frequently throughout the day, stop what you are doing and observe what you are thinking. Observe yourself objectively. Notice if your thoughts are helpful or unhelpful. Label them positive or negative.

2. When an unwanted thought arises and you want to release it and restore harmony in your mind, pause in what you are doing.

3. Take slow deep breaths, flushing your system with oxygen to lower your level of anxiety. Pay attention to your breath. You will soon reach a relaxed, helpful state called the "alpha" state, when your brain waves shift from an alert beta rhythm to a relaxed alpha rhythm.

4. Think about a pleasant scene: a mountain lake, a beach, any favored place of relaxation, or think about some upcoming event which you are looking forward to.

5. Practice this technique often throughout the day until you notice that the number of upsetting thoughts decreases.

If you find yourself repeatedly thinking the same unwanted thoughts, you might want to contemplate your reasons for having such thoughts and for wanting to change them. You may uncover something about yourself that you can change that will restore harmony to your thinking.

> *Until you make peace with who you are, you'll*
> *never be content with what you have.*
> —Doris Mortman

Sticks and stones can break my bones, but names can never harm me.

Think before you speak.

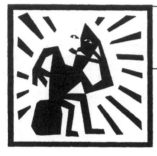

Chapter 3

How We Think and Talk About Disease

James Lance, in the book *Headache: Understanding Alleviation*, provides us with a poignant example of the body's response to words. "The dramatic term whiplash injury conjures up a vision of the patient's neck being cracked like a whip—imagery more vivid than is usually warranted by the circumstances. The very use of the term may be enough to make the patient retract his neck like a tortoise, causing the neck muscles to contract continuously, a potent cause of headache in its own right."[30]

Names as Symbols Evoke Images

The power of a name lies in its ability to evoke an image. Mention the name of a loved one and a set of feelings, thoughts, and images appear—perhaps many conflicting images. Mention the name of a place and a different set of feelings and thoughts arise. Mention the name of a disease like cancer or acne and still another set of images occur, perhaps accompanied by strong negative feelings. Negative feelings include worries, fears, depressions, jealousies, and hates, among others. Since they teach us about ourselves, they aren't bad. But left untended, these feelings can lead to illness.

The names of things matter because the images they evoke shape our thoughts and feelings, which in turn affect our bodies. As we name a thing we are also, in a sense, causing or creating it. The name reminds us of a previously encoded image that our body can then re-create. Expectation plays a major role. In obvious examples, placing the labels "heartbroken" or "heart sick" or even "sick to death of" on an emotional response can cause actual physical distress.

We have a tendency to want to name everything that happens to us. To avoid the ambiguity of not knowing and not understanding, we tend to label uncomfortable bodily states. Naming a set of symptoms often brings relief because people generally assume that knowing the name means something can be done about the illness. The name of a disease is important in planning treatment, so finding the right name is necessary. The diagnosis thus leads to treatment to relieve the unwanted condition. However, the name can also evoke unwanted images and expectations. These negatively influence the disease process, stressing an already strained body.

The label "cancer" causes fear in many people—even though the predicted outcome of a bout with cancer continues to improve. For many, cancer still feels like a death sentence. Tuberculosis had the same effect on people in the nineteenth century. When cancer was viewed as a sure death sentence, the patient often gave up hope. Today this former certainty has changed. Though many people still die of cancer and survival rates vary depending on the type of cancer, most cancer patients have reason to hope.

Currently, HIV Positive and AIDS are "label of death" words for most people invoking terror, because it is still often said that a fatal outcome from AIDS is inevitable. In 1990 AIDS was considered hopeless by almost everyone, despite some early evidence to the contrary. As early as 1986, Carolyn Reuben had written in *East West Journal* that many AIDS patients remained in remission, living years beyond the expectations of their doctors. But this was rarely talked about because, as Reuben wrote, "The belief system is so strong in our society that they will die. By saying you're in remission everybody who doesn't believe it's possible and thinks it's only temporary and you will die projects the thought form at you. You have to be a really strong individual."[31]

The March 1989 edition of *Brain/Mind Bulletin* had an article about an AIDS symposium at which ten long-term AIDS survivors spoke on a panel. Death from AIDS even then was not inevitable. Several AIDS patients who had survived years longer than expected even appeared on television. All of them "changed their minds" as part of their healing process. One woman who appeared on "The Phil Donohue Show" on June 20, 1989 said that three years prior, she had ARC—AIDS Related Complex. By 1989 she was well, with no signs of disease; she tested free of the HIV virus.

In 1996, ten years after Carolyn Reuben's *East West Journal* article on AIDS, a major shift in thinking had begun to take hold. Andrew Sullivan wrote about it in his *New York Times Magazine Section* article *WHEN PLAGUES END: Notes On The Twilight Of An Epidemic*. Though many still "find it hard to accept that this ordeal as a whole may be over... The power of the new treatments is such that a diagnosis of HIV infection ... no longer signifies death. It merely signifies illness."[32]

Not only that, but currently one need not panic even if one is exposed to an AIDS infected needle. According to Bridgeport, Connecticut, Gastroenterologist Dr. Ronald Levin M.D., "Now there is a medical protocol available that can prevent transmission of the HIV virus even after an accidental needle prick from a contaminated needle such as might occur under emergency room conditions. The preventive protocol currently involves a short [several days] course of treatment with a 3 drug 'anti AIDS cocktail'. Immediate treatment with these highly potent drugs will prevent any HIV virus transmitted from being able to replicate, multiply and take root. The key is speedy recognition of the exposure."[33]

Fortunately new treatments to suppress the replication of the HIV virus and better treatments for AIDS itself, mean that soon the label won't lead to the hopeless feeling that often insures a negative end result. Doctors, who are the purveyors of the name for a set of symptoms, can influence a patient's expectations by presenting the diagnosis in a framework of hope. Today there is hope for a person newly diagnosed HIV positive, though preventive measures to avoid contagion remain the prudent course of action for anyone uninfected.

Often only some of the symptoms of a particular disease are present at the time that a label is attached to an illness. The patient might then *expect* the missing symptoms to occur. Or, for instance, the physician might ask the patient whether he or she is experiencing other expected symptoms, presenting a subtle suggestion to the patient's mind.

Paul Pearsall in *Superimmunity* reports making the terrible mistake of asking one of his pregnant counseling patients, "Have you had morning sickness yet?" She responded that she was feeling just fine, "I can't believe how good the pregnancy is going." The next day she called Pearsall to report spending most of the night experiencing nausea. She concluded, "I really have it now."[34] Pearsall recognized that asking the question was probably a stimulus for his client's response.

Expectations often generate the unwanted result. However, not everyone gets every symptom of a particular disease or condition, just as lots of women, myself included, never experience morning sickness when they are pregnant. On the contrary, give a person the proper physical, mental, and emotional support and the body can cure just about any condition.

The Advent of the *Sinus Headache*

When a particular set of feelings and behaviors—"symptoms"—are grouped together and named, a new disease emerges. The identification of the disease called AIDS led to the research that is defining the actions necessary to control and someday even cure it. But sometimes less positively, naming a set of symptoms generates new victims.

In communication theory, the Sapir-Whorf hypothesis states: When you have a name for something, you are much more likely to perceive it. The classic example is that of the Eskimos. They have dozens of words for different kinds of snow, and they see all those different kinds. Those of us who live in more temperate climates have only one word for snow, with a few variations, so that one kind of snow is all we generally perceive.

John Bear, Ph.D., told me the following story, which illustrates the above effect:

"The notion that you feel, experience, and suffer from things for which you have words became clear to me in the early 60's. At a big New York advertising agency, I met a man famous in the annals of advertising because he had invented a disease. You see, when a new drug comes along, it requires years of testing before the Food and Drug Administration (FDA) approves it. This man's stroke of genius was to take an already approved drug—one that was languishing in sales—and invent a new disease that the drug could help. New diseases do not have to be approved by the FDA!

"The drug in question was Dristan, then a modestly-selling cold and headache remedy. This man invented the name 'sinus headache.' He named a collection of symptoms which were then recognized as a new disease. He used language to distinguish this as an entirely new headache. Actually, people had probably often suffered head pain from sinus distress without knowing why. Now they knew! This advertising genius then wrote a whole series of advertisements presenting Dristan as the only product that could cure a sinus headache. All over America, people suddenly started having sinus headaches in ever increasing numbers, propelling Dristan onto the bestseller list of over-the-counter remedies. Nearly 20 years later, the sinus headache has become a standard ailment which even appears in some medical texts. Such is the power of language in creating disease."[35]

Anorexia and Bulimia

Much attention has been focused on the eating disorders called anorexia and bulimia. There were some people engaging in anorexic and bulimic behaviors who didn't know they had a disease until they heard the names and learned what they represented. Long before I knew the word "bulimia," an acquaintance introduced me to the idea of vomiting to control weight—although it never appealed to me personally. Perhaps anorexic and bulimic behaviors seem more prevalent now, because they have been named and well-publicized. Sometimes, naming a set of symptoms encourages others who have the illness to come forward. The identification of anorexia and bulimia as distinct syndromes led to successful treatments.

However, it is possible that many people have been falsely labeled "anorexic." I have wondered about several friends who are very thin. Attaching labels to people is dangerous since people have a tendency to become what we expect of them. On the other hand, perhaps the fear of anorexia will help release some people addicted to the idea that only thin is beautiful.

Does the name of a disease, like "sinus headache" or "anorexia" help people to feel less alone by naming the symptoms they are experiencing and the behaviors they are engaged in? Does the name encourage them to seek treatment? Or does the name plant an idea in their consciousness, encouraging some people to adopt the behaviors and develop the symptoms? Which comes first, the name or the disease?

Copy Cat Disease Syndrome

We are familiar with the copycat crime syndrome in which unusual crimes, when reported in the media, cause a rash of similar crimes. In the same way there may be a copycat disease syndrome. A classic example of this occurred many years ago in Los Angeles. During a game at Monterey Park Football Stadium, several people began experiencing symptoms of food poisoning. Soft drinks from a particular machine were the suspected cause. An announcement was broadcast over the stadium public address system warning patrons that drinks from such a machine could cause severe nausea and other symptoms. Soon, hundreds of people began exhibiting similar symptoms of food poisoning. Many were even hospitalized for observation. Shortly thereafter, it was announced that the soft drink machine was not involved in the food poisoning. Immediately people's symptoms began to clear.

People tend to imitate the behavior of others. When they hear of certain behaviors, this at least implants the idea that such behaviors are possible, a possibility that might never have otherwise occurred to them. This could be significant in relation to anxiety diseases like phobias. Some people develop phobias after hearing about them. The same could be said about any of the compulsive disease disorders.

We've all heard the expression *sympathy pains*. Research into the lives of husbands of pregnant women indicates that some husbands exhibit many of the sensations and behaviors associated with pregnancy, like food cravings and morning sickness. When you describe an action, even a dysfunctional one, you can reinforce the idea of engaging in that action. Medical students are known to often exhibit the symptoms of diseases they are studying. These imitations may not be common, but they do occur. Ideas implanted in a receptive mind have power to help or hurt.

On the other hand, people often seek treatment after hearing or reading about a disease. Television is a major source of information about all manner of unusual conditions. From the evening news, 20/20, Dateline and 60 Minutes to the broad range of Cable TV shows, from Oprah, Montel, Sally Jessy and other talk shows to the Movie of the Week, we learn about medical oddities, rarities and dysfunctional behaviors. These less well-known conditions, such as Self-Mutilation, Agoraphobia, Compulsive Disorder Syndrome, or Severe Obesity, may afflict hundreds or more viewers. Often, they first heard about the disease, and possible treatments, from television. Sometimes, these people hadn't even realized they were suffering from a named disease and that a cure is possible using a defined treatment plan.

More recently, going "on-line" to surf the Internet and World Wide Web has become a powerful method for networking and locating self-help information regarding diagnosis and treatment. As more of us get online we share all manner of information related to disease. *Please remember to get professional advice before attempting self treatment recommended by these or any other sources.* Nevertheless, one can benefit enormously from sharing information.

Hypertension

Hypertension—high blood pressure—is a disease that seems to be related to feelings of powerlessness. Hypertension has been studied extensively for many years. In the 1980's John Sommers-Flanagan of the University of Montana and Roger Greenberg of the State University of New York reviewed forty-eight empirical studies which linked hypertension with various psychological factors. They found evidence of three primary psychological characteristics of hypertensives:

1. Anger/hostility.
2. Difficulty with interpersonal contact and communication.
3. Frequent use of denial and self-repression.

They also found that the traditional treatment for hypertension typically includes drugs, exercise, and diet. As a result of their 1980's research, Sommers-Flanagan and Greenberg recommended that psychological approaches be used more often to supplement, or even replace, traditional medical solutions. Greenberg said, "We felt that the part personality plays has been increasingly undervalued. There seems to have been a trend toward regarding many disorders as exclusively biological. We think an integrated approach is necessary."[36]

Psychosocial intervention could enhance the ability of hypertension patients to control the physical effects of their tension-provoking experiences by reducing anxiety and increasing coping skills. In 1996, Connecticut Cardiologist Steven Kunkes M.D. who has long provided me with needed information and support told me, "Lifestyle changes are being emphasized more often now for hypertension patients."[37]

Thomas Pickering, M.D.[38], reported that men employed in jobs combining high work demands with a low level of perceived control over their work environment have increased blood pressure throughout the day and night, not just during working hours. Several studies have indicated that blood pressure may be higher in people for whom there is a mismatch between their environment and their aspirations (e.g., those with "champagne tastes on a beer budget") These studies seem to indicate that lifestyle changes, including changes in attitude and underlying thought patterns, will be helpful in controlling hypertension.

Dr. Robban Sica confirmed the efficacy of helping patients to make lifestyle changes. She explained to me, "I have many patients with labile or fluctuating hypertension. In such cases, it is clear that a variety of factors are affecting them, everything from obesity, a diet containing excessive carbohydrates, deficiency of minerals such as magnesium or potassium, to job, financial, or relationship stress, to fearful thoughts, unproductive worrying, and feeling a lack of control in life. In addition to nutritional intervention, weight loss, and exercise, I educate them medically about helpful stress reduction techniques such as meditation and the benefits of changing limiting thoughts about their ability to change their own life."[39]

Connecticut specialist in pulmonary and internal medicine, Dr. David Bushell M.D. agreed, "I think stress reduction techniques have a positive physiological function and are useful adjunctive treatments for many ailments. It's pretty clear that stress reduction techniques for hypertension in particular are now recommended by a large number of doctors."[40]

The Grammar of Disease

While diagnosing and naming a disease can be very useful in the healing process, some of the negative effects of naming are less obvious. Names are always nouns. Naming a disease as a noun reinforces the idea that anorexia, arthritis, cancer, heart attack, hypertension, strep throat and whiplash are events that "just happen to us" and which we cannot control or be responsible for. This use of language reinforces a view of ourselves as victims of the events in our lives. Now we have a particular event which we call a "disease," and we have given it a name. Such language diminishes our feeling of being in control of our lives. Feeling a lack of control has itself been linked to the progress of disease.

Where labels for people are concerned, calling a person an "alcoholic" or a "drug addict" can be either positive or negative: positive if it helps a person take actions that move them away from that illness; negative if the person feels and continues to act like a victim, stuck forever with diseased behavior. The label can also create an image in the mind of others which may reinforce the victim's unwanted behavior patterns. The expectations of others can influence our thoughts, our choice of words, our actions and our negative behaviors.

The old adage, "Sticks and stones can break my bones, but names can never harm me" is incorrect. Call someone stupid or lazy and the label can stick, becoming a self-fulfilling prophecy. See someone as an alcoholic, or a sugar junkie, and you might be feeding their disease. However, you might also be identifying what's wrong with them, leading them to seek help.

In the ongoing, ever-changing drama of health, *psyche* (the mind and emotions) and *soma* (the body) engage in a variety of behaviors sometimes called symptoms. We give meaning to the behaviors, such as good or bad, positive or negative, healthy or sick, well or diseased. We often give the behavior the name of a specific disease. *But dis-ease is a human behavioral process, not just a specific entity with a label and a definition.* The label is merely a convenient way to describe a set of symptoms the ill person experiences. I sometimes hyphenate dis-ease to indicate that when I'm not feeling well, I'm not at ease within myself, that my mind, body, and emotions are out of sync. *Disease* is the opposite of being *at ease*.

The following statements illustrate how we usually talk about sickness:

"I'm getting a cold."

"My child caught chicken pox."

"Jane has AIDS."

"I had an allergy attack."

"He has pimples."

All the above examples presuppose disease as something external to us, an invader that is not part of us, something that comes from somewhere else and imposes itself upon us for a time. Something external to us may indeed trigger the disease, but it is *our* body that reacts.

These common expressions and various labels are useful, often making it unnecessary to describe the symptoms being experienced. But this way of talking also helps us to feel like victims and contributes to our avoiding taking personal responsibility for our health. People who continue to feel like victims often do nothing to help themselves. A responsible person takes action to eliminate the dis-ease.

The grammatical structure of the language of disease thus suggests that we play no major part in causing an illness. Yet the labels we use to name things have a great deal to do with how we see things. Naming the disease with a noun often conveys the impression that the illness is an invasion of our body by an enemy entity rather than an on-going dis-easing process in which we are fully engaged. When disease is seen as external to ourselves, something we catch or get, we convey the impression that measles, cancer, or acne are conditions over which we have no control. Perhaps we have more control than we know.

If you are obese, saying "I overeat" allows you to recognize yourself as the source of your overweight condition. Once this point of inner control is established, you can choose to change the amount and type of food you eat and your level of physical activity. These changes do frequently lead to weight loss and a release from the obesity (a noun) behavior pattern. You can also change your mind about what you think of as fat and release yourself from any negative self-judgments. Recognizing your role in creating dis-ease improves your chances of releasing the dis-ease and returning to good health.

In the case of illness triggered by something outside ourselves such as a specific bacteria or virus, we note that not everyone exposed to such things gets sick. Illness comes from how you talk and what you think and feel, among other causes. An immune system able to withstand the effects of outside forces may well be a function of our underlying thoughts, feelings and attitudes. And whether or not a foreign organism actually makes our bodies ill may be subject to our conscious control.

Ancient Wisdom of the Power of Words

Knowledge of the power of the spoken word dates back to the ancient world. From the Bible we learn that God created the world through sound using the power of speech. Starting in Genesis Chapter One Verse 3 we read, "*God said:* Let there be light." In successive verses *God speaks* the whole earth and its inhabitants into existence. We too use sound and words in the process of creating our personal reality.

Later in Verse 27 of Genesis Chapter One we read "And God created man in his image." But what is meant by "in His image?" God appears to have had a vision in mind, and created humanity according to that vision. Human beings would then be an exact replica of God's visionary thoughtform just as a photograph is an exact replica of an image etched on a negative. God's image was first translated into words and then became flesh. This provides a clue for us as to the way we might envision and create our personal reality: *we can use our thoughts to envision and create health and happiness.*

How we think and speak about our lives and ourselves is a key component to living a quality life. The Christian Bible speaks of this in the book of James (Ch 3:3–7):

"If anyone can control his tongue, it proves that he has perfect control over himself in every other way. We can make a large horse turn around and go wherever we want by means of a small bit in his mouth. And a tiny rudder makes a huge ship turn wherever the pilot wants it to go, even though the winds are strong. So also the tongue is a small thing, but what enormous damage it can do. A great forest can be set on fire by one tiny spark. And the tongue is a flame of fire. It is full of wickedness, and poisons every part of the body. And the tongue is set on fire by hell itself, and can turn our whole lives into a blazing flame of destruction and disaster."[41]

Judaism too has lots to say about the power of the tongue. For example, "The tongue is like an arrow. If a person raises a sword to kill his fellow and then changes his mind, he can return the sword to its scabbard. But the arrow, once it has been fired cannot be called back."[42] Ancient wisdom on the power of words is valuable information. Recently a woman wrote:

"Just before the sudden death of my spiritual advisor his enemies often said 'We wish you would drop dead'. His wife told me, 'Allen felt heart-broken over those stressful events in our community. As one of Allen's strongest and most outspoken supporters in the congregation, I too caught a lot of the flack. I was devastated, my heart stricken with grief and pain when this great leader, a hero who fell on the battlefield, a champion of human rights and social justice died of a sudden and massive heart attack. My friends were all shocked when I resigned from the congregation about this time, because I'd been so actively involved in it for so long. But quite frankly, it had become so stressful that I do believe it would have been the death of me too if I'd stayed."[43]

Words too, like bullets once fired, may do irreparable damage which can affect more people than they originally were intended to hurt. Just like a gust of wind can blow down a tower of cards, some ill-chosen words can wreak unbelievable havoc.

Your Power to Influence Your Health

You may not want to recognize yourself as the source of your ailments. But until you do, you are not in the driver's seat and cannot begin to *think of yourself as the source of healing as well: you caused it, to some degree, and you can uncause it, to the same degree.* There is no self-blame intended in this statement. There are factors involved in any illness over which you have little, if any, control. Nevertheless, you can perceive or recognize that you do have some power over your health via your thoughts, your attitudes, your words, your actions and your behaviors.

It is important to accept yourself and learn from past mistakes, rather than cause yourself more dis-ease by feelings of self-hate and guilt. Most health professionals would agree: *Loving yourself is an important component in healing.* A spiritual teacher once told me, "Love yourself fully and then you can love everyone else. Take care of yourself, so you can take care of everyone else." Maybe that's the true meaning of the biblical command to love your neighbor as yourself. First, we have to learn how to love ourselves.

Disease is not a thing that happens to you; it is a way of acting out life. You are responsible for everything in your life, whether you believe it or not. When you recognize this truth you will begin to accept that *you are in charge of your health at the subtle level of thoughts and words as well as the obvious level of actions.* Granted, altering the effects of past thoughts and actions might take quite a while. The process might even seem to be irrevocable if it has gone on for years. But people quite often experience miraculous cures even from so-called incurable or terminal diseases. Responsibility fosters hope, and that often leads to self-induced healing. We can train ourselves to think thoughts and use words that will lead to health rather than illness.

Self-Help Experience #5

Is "Cancer" a Verb?

Purpose: To increase your sense of control over your body.

We name diseases with nouns. But since disease is actually a behavioral process we engage in, try using the disease name as a verb. Verbs are process words indicating some action you take. As a semantic exercise, try changing the noun for acne or cancer to a verb.

Say: "I am acne-ing," not "I have acne." "My body is cancer-ing," not "I have cancer." It may be awkward to talk in this way, but which way of talking implies greater personal control?

Use the name of your illness as a verb to indicate that illness as an ongoing process which you act out. See if you feel more responsible for what ails you. *Being responsible does not mean blaming yourself.* Being responsible does mean accepting yourself and then doing what is appropriate to help yourself—be it taking medicine or acting in new ways.

> *Disease can be healed if we are willing to change the way we think and believe and act.*
> —Louise Hay

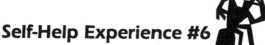

Self-Help Experience #6

Questions Concerning Catastrophic Illness

Purpose: To increase the patient's self-knowledge during illness; to discover the patient's basic attitudes toward being healed.

The following are key questions to ask oneself, or another, at the onset or upon diagnosis of a catastrophic illness. The self-knowledge gained from the answers can motivate the patient toward recovery.

After much self-reflection, one woman recognized that she

broke her leg so she wouldn't have to continue a teaching job in a school she "couldn't stand." She couldn't quit because she was "supporting" her husband in dental school. Instead, she broke her leg skiing. She said, "The broken leg got me out of teaching. Because I wasn't capable of moving fast in the event of a school fire, I had 'no choice' but to stop. But the price of the 'accident' was heavy. It took six months for my leg to heal and much of that time I was stuck in the house."

Before answering each question, close your eyes, relax, and look deeply within your heart and soul to find the truth. Take time to contemplate each question. Be wary of automatic answers.

1. *How long do you want to live?*

Do you love yourself enough to take care of your mind and body? Do you look forward to the future with hope or fear? These questions help you to uncover your will to live and how much control you feel you have in life.

2. *What happened in the year or two before your illness?* List those experiences, both positive and negative, that had a major impact on you. Examples: getting married or divorced, death of a loved one, getting a new job or being fired, starting or losing a business.

3. *What does the illness mean to you?* Do you consider it an automatic death sentence? Some people expect to live, no matter what the odds. Others expect to die no matter what the odds. You are an individual who has the power to control how you feel and how you heal. You can beat the odds either way.

4. *Why do you need this illness?* Since sickness often gives people permission to avoid things they really don't want to do, or to do things they wouldn't permit themselves to do, this is a key question to ask for any illness, major or minor. People get sick to take time off from their usual ways of behaving. A bout with colds or flu might be avoided if people took more "personal" days off from work, rather than "sickness days." The sickness allows them to escape their "shoulds." "I should do this...be this...feel this way."

Watch out for emergencies. They are your big chance.
—Fritz Reiner

Roll over and play dead.

Don't bite off more than you can chew.

Chapter 4

Responsibility and Creative Intelligence

The guiding light of the body is the mind. Recognizing the connection between language and health enables you to expand control of your health process. This language connection consists of the thoughts, words, imaginings, mental pictures, and emotions that stimulate illness and wellness. By correctly using your language connection, *dis-easing* behavior can be transformed so that you can be healed. Behavior includes actions, lifestyle, thoughts, and spoken words.

You may feel like a victim of this body process (disease), since most symptoms (body behaviors) are not consciously induced. Take pimples, for example: you choose to ignore, squeeze, or medicate a pimple, but you don't consciously choose to have one. During a cold, your body secretes mucus, your nose runs, you sneeze and cough. You can choose to blow your nose, but you aren't aware of choosing to have the excess mucus. Something in you, however, is causing the pimple to erupt or the mucus to secrete. With cancer, cell division runs amok, though the conscious part of your mind wouldn't choose cancering behavior.

Who or what is controlling these body behaviors? How does it know what to do? Can you guide the inner intelligence that controls the automatic functions and behaviors of your body? Is it possible to gain some control over this creative process and choose your level of health or illness? To a large degree, the answer is "Yes." *Dis-ease is a process over which you can have more control by carefully choosing your thoughts, your words, your attitude, and your actions.* When you are responsible, you have the choice of altering the way that you think, speak, and act in order to change the effects. Using healthful rather than harmful words, you are taking responsibility for your healthy functioning. Your creative intelligence is now operating in your behalf, rather than to your detriment.

We face many choices in the course of a lifetime. We may not always be able to choose our circumstances, but we have freedom to choose how we feel about those circumstances. We can choose to be upset, despairing, angry, and envious—or happy, satisfied, and content. We can ignore our feelings or listen to them and learn from them. Free choice means that we realize we have the choice.

Meaning and Reality

Viktor Frankl, M.D., sheds light on the choices we each can make in *Man's Search for Meaning*. The book, a moving account of his incarceration in various Nazi concentration camps during World War II, also presents the basic concepts of Logotherapy—a psychotherapy he developed and later refined as a result of those harrowing years in the camps. He wrote:

"The experiences of camp life show that man does have a choice of action. There were enough examples, often of a heroic nature, which proved that apathy could be overcome, irritability suppressed. Man *can* preserve a vestige of spiritual freedom, of independence of mind, even in such terrible conditions of psychic and physical stress.

"We who lived in concentration camps can remember the men who walked through the huts comforting others, giving away their last piece of bread. They may have been few in number, but they offer sufficient proof that *everything can be taken from a man but one thing: the last of the human freedoms—to choose one's attitude in any given set of circumstances, to choose one's own way.* In the final analysis it becomes clear that the sort of person the prisoner became was the result of an inner decision, and not the result of camp influences alone. Fundamentally therefore, any man can, even under such circumstances, decide what shall become of him—mentally and spiritually."[44]

Dr. Wallace C. Ellerbroek was for many years a prominent California surgeon, psychiatrist, and amateur psycholinguist. After years of informal research and a formal research project using acne patients, he realized that *disease arises not so much out of what happens to us but as a result of how we see things, and the things we tell ourselves.* He once wrote, "It isn't what happens that bugs you, it's the things that you say in your head about what happens that makes all the machinery get messed up, and leads to varieties of disease."[45]

Dr. Ellerbroek tested his theory of disease on a group of thirty-eight acne patients, aged 13 to 46. Acne patients "pick at" their lesions and they frequently feel "picked on" in life. His patients generally interpreted anything they did not like as abuse aimed personally at them. His thesis was that the acne would improve if the "picked on" thought pattern and other contributory behavior could be decreased or eliminated. He treated them with a combination of psychological and psycholinguistic therapy designed to change the patients' thinking so they no longer felt like victims. Based on subjective observations by himself and the patients, the results were excellent. Of the thirty-eight original patients, thirty were judged 80 percent improved within eight weeks. Over a longer period of time, more than half of the patients achieved clear skin. The remainder showed 80–90 percent improvement. Here is how Dr. Ellerbroek explained his results:

"We humans create mental pictures of what we observe in the external world, our version of reality. This evaluation of reality is often inaccurate, due to limitations of our sensory organs and inadequate mechanisms for verifying our perceptions. At any given moment we have a personal idea of how we think the past, present, and future *should* be. Reality can be seen as the way we want it to be, the way we *think* it really is, or the way it *actually* is.

"When our world seems to match our picture of how we think it should be, we feel good. When humans become aware that their version of reality doesn't match their fantasy of how it should be, they often irrationally and unconsciously demand that reality be changed to match their fantasy. The failure of reality to alter itself to match their fantasy can lead to depression and frustration, the emotions that are the core of illness.

"An example of this unrealistic demand is reflected in the negative emotions felt when we think life isn't going our way. Perhaps the weather spoiled a picnic or an employee called in sick and we must do the extra work. In our fantasy-reality these things are not okay occurrences. To the extent that we deny the validity of these events, we will experience the upsetting emotions that in turn often cause illness. Yet what happened has already happened and can't be changed.

"Years spent treating patients as a psychiatrist and surgeon convinced me that mental and physical illness are different manifestations of the same disease process: negative thinking. Your brain is patterned by everything that happens throughout your life, even back to the moment you were conceived. So all the years you were, for example, thinking picked-on thoughts, your brain was recording these. Since we all tend to continue doing whatever we do, it becomes obvious that learning a new process of thinking is not an easy or trivial thing to do. I am also convinced, from my years in practice, that effective treatment is attainable."[46]

From Resistance to Acceptance of Reality

The Holocaust—the murder by the Nazis of 6 million Jews along with countless millions of others—is probably the best documented atrocity in recorded history. Yet still, there exist revisionists who would deny altogether that the Holocaust even took place. These deniers are a prime example of people trying to make reality conform to their own desired picture. Some events are so horrifying that there are some people who won't ever face the truth.

Another example of people attempting to make reality conform to their preferred inner pictures occurred in China during the student revolt in Tienanmen Square. The Chinese Communist leadership attempted to cover up the violence committed by the government against their own people. Despite the whole world witnessing many of these events on TV, the leadership still attempted to convince us that what everyone knows happened didn't really happen. TV allows us to be eyewitnesses to history. It's been said, "I will believe it when I see it" and "there are none so blind as those that will not see." The underlying reality of these statements echoes the truth that *we often will see only what we already believe is possible.*

Acceptance of reality is the beginning of taking responsibility for your life. Often you can control events, but just as often you must adapt to circumstances beyond your control. How you adapt—the thoughts you think, the words you speak, and the attitude you take—determines your state of health and your chance of recovery. Thinking and speaking like a victim discourages healing. You change your experience by first recognizing the role your emotions, thoughts, and speech play in inducing disease.

A big part of your role is to envision and believe that healing is possible. Hope helps! Loss of hope is deadly! Your body's innate wisdom knows how to heal itself. But, it can also create the physical symptoms associated with despair, or any other emotional attitude.

Even cases of so-called "terminal" cancer have been reversed. Psychotherapist Warren Berland studied 33 people who lived for an extended time period despite a "terminal" medical prognosis. He questioned, "Why do some patients with grim prognosis outlive their doctors' predictions for recovery or survival?"[47] He noted that "those studied were considerably more likely than the norm to attribute recovery to their own resources than to powerful others or to fate." From patients who survived and managed to improve the quality of their lives, Berland frequently heard, "Thank God I got cancer—I never could have or would have made these changes in my life."

From his study Berland concluded, "Participants gave almost twice the credit for their recovery to factors other than their medical treatment...There is no right way to heal...Some people focused their attention on fighting to survive. Others prayed, visualized, changed their attitude about themselves, and altered how they lived their lives... Some deepened their sense of meaning and purpose..."[48] Anyone stricken or afflicted with a life-threatening disease must keep in mind the idea that they have the capacity to influence the outcome of their disease no matter what the generally expected prognosis. So-called re-markable, unexpected, often unexplainable recoveries happen more frequently than we realize.

As early as the late 1980's reports began to appear about long-time survivors of the usually deadly AIDS virus. An Advanced Immune Discoveries Symposium in Los Angeles featured a panel of ten long-term survivors.[49] AIDS patients and some long-term survivors have appeared on several TV talk shows, often bringing messages of hope. One man said he no longer tests positive for AIDS, although he had had several bouts with AIDS symptoms—pneumonia and cancer. A woman in the audience who had been diagnosed with Aids Related Complex (ARC) was also now virus free. ARC was then considered the pre-cursor to fullblown AIDS.

By February 1997, it was widely reported by the Centers For Disease Control, that for the first time ever, there had been a 13% decline in death rates from AIDS. Then in June 1998 an article in the New York Times Magazine reported on what "scientists had known for some time about a small group of people they call long-term nonprogressors." These people "suppress the virus without ever taking drugs."[50]

Furthermore there were instances reported of patients whose own immune system had taken back the role of suppressing the Aids-causing virus after "early aggressive treatment." This led researchers to posit that "early aggressive treatment might transform ordinary patients into long-term nonprogressors who don't need drugs to contain HIV." Some people had stopped taking their drugs yet remained essentially virus and symptom free.

In seeking to understand how the patient's own immune system can reclaim its disease-fighting function, the attitude of the patient appears to play a significant part. It seems clear that the old adage, *where there's a will there's a way*, is true. We are making real progress in healing or alleviating even this most severe disease.

Ronald Glasser, M.D. writes, "It is the body that is the hero, not science, not antibiotics...not machines or new devices....The task of the physician today is what it has always been, to help the body do what it has learned so well to do on its own during its unending struggle for survival—to heal itself. It is the body, not medicine, that is the hero."[51] To this I might add, it is the body directed by a conscious creative mind which is most likely to recover.

Your language affects your body both positively and negatively. When you think about situations that make you angry, your blood pressure can rise. Some people get red in the face. Often the heart beats faster and the jaws clench. These physical reactions are caused by thoughts which trigger emotions and vice versa. Emotions trigger more thoughts as you give meaning to what you feel. This vicious, self-reinforcing cycle, if it becomes a habit, will eventually bring itself graphically to your attention as physical symptoms. A feeling is the physical manifestation of emotional energy. Happy thoughts promote healing! A smile or a hearty laugh are stress reducers. Pay attention to those thoughts which promote your well-being and those which make you feel rotten.

Obviously how you feel affects your thoughts and words. When you feel head pain you say, "I have a headache." Less obviously, the process also works in reverse: *what you think and say affects how you feel.* Frustrated over work, you might say, "This project is one big headache." Later your head may actually begin to hurt. You meant to express frustration about the difficulty of a project, not invite pain in. However, your body, run by your unconscious mind, might not understand that you are speaking metaphorically. Your unconscious mind can create an unwanted condition in your body by taking your statements quite literally. At the cellular level, the mind does not understand what you really meant. The mind/body system cannot distinguish fact from metaphor.

Unconscious and Conscious Awareness

Your mind, an innate intelligence, connects intimately to your body by organizing your inner life and controlling automatic body functions. It serves you in planning and remembering and so on. You don't have to think about breathing, or secreting digestive enzymes, or producing immune system cells, although you can put your attention on these things and, for example, consciously choose to breathe slower or faster, like a Lamaze patient in the throes of labor. But much of the time, it's just as well to let the part of mind that operates the body run itself automatically. Although we often speak of an unconscious mind and a conscious/aware mind, that implies a separation that does not in fact exist. These terms are chosen simply for linguistic convenience, since there is just one mind that operates the body.

The part of your mind that thinks, reasons, and makes choices is where consciousness or awareness is most desirable. But, even here, your mind is not always conscious of its work. Your so-called conscious mind changes as you choose to pay attention. You engage in selective awareness. Just as a child engrossed in a TV show might not hear his mother calling him, you will not notice all the work—the thoughts and feelings—of your own mind. Similarly, your so-called unconscious mind expands or contracts as formerly unconscious processes surface and reach a level where you notice them, just as mom's yelling or turning the TV off causes her child to pay attention and get the message.

The so-called unconscious mind is that part of your mind whose contents you are unaware of at any given time. Sometimes this is to your benefit: you don't have to think about all the millions of automatic processes needed to keep you functioning. You don't tell your digestive enzymes to flow or stop to think about breathing. Your internal operating system (akin to the disk operating system on a personal computer) handles this very well. Sometimes to your detriment unconscious material influences your choices and leads to negative behaviors. For example, if you are angry at your spouse and unable to admit your feelings, you might do something to undermine him—perhaps spill a glass of soda on him accidentally on purpose. In such a case, you may really believe it was an accident, yet some part of you needed to act out in order to express your feelings.

The human body is a network of billions of interconnected cells, each in communication with the others but mostly beneath your conscious awareness. You, as creative awareness, reside in that body. The body is the temple of the spirit, the house of the soul, and the reflection of the mind. Put another way: Your body is the temple of the Living God. Each cell, through a spark of consciousness, knows how to re-create and program itself. The intelligence within each cell is considered to be part of your unconscious, non-reasoning mind. When these cells receive a message about a headache, they can join together to create an ache in your head. In this sense, language becomes a connecting link among the cells in your body.

Psychologist Dr. Dennis Jaffe, writing in *Healing From Within* asks a key question, "Are specific diseases related to particular life crises, personality types or emotions?" He continues, "though I have studiously avoided proclaiming this connection as a reflection of reality, physicians have detected a link between emotions, personality, and specific illness for centuries. A growing number of recent studies have added support to this hypothesis."[52] Jaffe came to this conclusion after studying the work of psychosomatic experts W.J. Grace and D.T. Graham.[53] Jaffe wrote:

"Grace and Graham had conducted in-depth interviews with one hundred twenty-eight patients, each of whom had the symptoms of one of twelve different diseases. The researchers were trying to determine what life-situations were associated with attacks of the patients' symptoms. Certain emotional attitudes, they found, were related to the onset of symptoms of each specific disease. They speculated that, in effect, the patients were expressing physiologically what they felt was being done to them in their every day lives.

"For example, twenty-seven patients reported attacks of diarrhea when they wanted to end a particular situation, or to get rid of something or somebody. One man developed this symptom after purchasing a defective automobile, telling the researchers, 'If only I could get rid of it.' Defecation, of course, is ridding oneself of substances after the body is done with them.

"Another seventeen patients had constipation when they were grimly determined to persevere through a seemingly insurmountable problem. They used statements such as, 'This marriage is never going to be any better, but I won't quit.' And what is constipation but a bodily process of holding on to substances without change, despite discomfort?

"Twelve patients with hay fever and seven with asthma articulated another set of attitudes. They faced a situation that they would rather not have had to confront, or that they wished would disappear. They wanted to hide from it, avoid it and divest themselves from all responsibility for it. Grace and Graham noted that these two syndromes—asthma and hay fever—often occurred together. They are both reactions to an external irritant in which the membranes of the nose and lungs swell up and narrow, in their attempt to dilute the irritant or wash it away. The body, just like the person, wants to get rid of something.

"Thirty one patients suffered from urticaria, a skin reaction to trauma, leading to blistering and inflammation. The patients with this ailment felt they were being interfered with or prevented from doing something they wanted to do. And they could not find a way to deal effectively with their frustration. They were so preoccupied with the way that others interfered with them that it was as if they were being physically beaten by their adversaries—hence the skin blisters.

"Nausea and vomiting (in eleven patients) occurred when a person wished something had never occurred. Ulcers (nine patients) were characterized by desires for revenge and getting even. Migraine headaches (fourteen patients) were provoked after a person had made an intense effort to complete a task. Hypertension was common among those who continually worried about meeting all possible threats (Type A behavior). Low back pain (eleven patients) was found among people who wanted to do something involving the whole body, usually running away."

This study dramatically supports the idea that your emotions can translate into body language, especially if you don't admit or act on your feelings. Note the resemblances with Ellerbroek's patients, who felt picked on, and *literally picked on themselves as well*. The feelings remain hidden, perhaps even from you, until they manifest in some illness. People sometimes push themselves into disease in order to express their unacknowledged emotions. Of course, they don't generally realize that they are doing this.

Getting the Message Through Disease

Physical sensations such as itching, crying, rashes, sweating, pain, pressure, orgasm, and smiles are all part of the language of the body. So is disease. During illness the body communicates whether our actions are detracting from or adding to our well-being.

Milton Ward, in a wonderfully helpful book entitled *The Brilliant Function Of Pain*, wrote "Pain, rather than being a terror, is actually our own brilliant force, functioning in our behalf, ready to guide us through life if we are but willing to listen.[54] Pain transmits a powerful message from body to mind. In this way it serves to communicate the way to health. Disease is your body's way of talking to you, telling you that something isn't working, showing you graphically and sometimes painfully that something is amiss.

When you are "diseasing," your body is actually attempting to heal itself by correcting imbalances and restoring harmony. *Feeling bad is often the route to getting better.* During acneing, for example, the skin pushes out toxins that aren't removed through the primary channels of elimination. A cold eliminates excess mucus, an effect of poor eating, environmental pressures, and other stresses and strains on the body. Even the rash of chicken pox contains toxic, contagious material that the body is eliminating. A tumor is your body's attempt to encapsulate cells grown awry. Perhaps your body doesn't have the strength to eliminate this threat any other way.

Life-threatening and chronic degenerative illnesses can result from negative thoughts and feelings, among other known causes. Yet disease, rather than an event to be feared, is frequently a positive force enabling us to see what changes are necessary to improve ourselves. We make the necessary changes by taking charge of our behaviors. We take charge when we realize that we act out through disease our conscious and unconscious beliefs and thought patterns. When we look at our illness and other crises in the context of this larger picture we can grow spiritually and emotionally.

Erik Esselstyn, Ed.D., who was then director of the Gesell Institute of Human Development in New Haven, was a guest speaker during one of my courses. During a bout with cancer, he faced his emotions and changed his thinking. When he got cancer Erik was dean of students at a college in North Carolina. The experience changed his career path.

Erik and his wife Micki, M.S.W, M.Div., led seminars and workshops on releasing anger and creating life changes because of major illness. Micki, as the "well spouse" around Erik's cancer was a spokesperson for the needs of the families of cancer patients. Micki said, "We have cancer to thank for a lot—it made us appreciate life." Erik said, "A key element in achieving and maintaining good health is the acceptance of personal responsibility for our own actions, gracefully acknowledging the fact that *each one of us is responsible for putting on his own seat belt."* [55]

We Are Not Victims

Many people aren't aware of their power to make themselves sick or to heal themselves. Your initial response to the idea that you cause your own disease might be skepticism, fear, anger, or dismay. Skepticism is reasonable. If your reaction is fear, anger, or dismay, it might be worthwhile to examine the source of your feelings. Perhaps you feel that way because you equate responsibility with blame and shame. You may not be used to forgiving yourself for your mistakes, changing to more appropriate behavior, and then forgetting about it. Some people think they have to act perfectly and when they don't, they punish and berate themselves with negative self-talk and feelings of guilt.

We are not victims. Rather, when we forget to take responsibility for our health, we often choose unconsciously to harm ourselves. Then we feel like victims of the fates. There is a better way of thinking available. But, it takes awareness and practice. You don't have to roll over and play dead. When you choose to be responsible for your own health and well-being, there is a lot you can do to help yourself. The aware use of the guiding light in your mind is a powerful way to help yourself to be well. You can train yourself to communicate health-producing thoughts so that your body becomes disease-free.

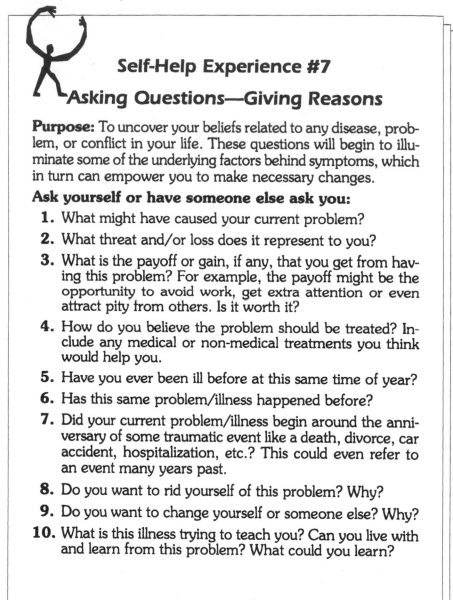

Self-Help Experience #7

Asking Questions—Giving Reasons

Purpose: To uncover your beliefs related to any disease, problem, or conflict in your life. These questions will begin to illuminate some of the underlying factors behind symptoms, which in turn can empower you to make necessary changes.

Ask yourself or have someone else ask you:

1. What might have caused your current problem?

2. What threat and/or loss does it represent to you?

3. What is the payoff or gain, if any, that you get from having this problem? For example, the payoff might be the opportunity to avoid work, get extra attention or even attract pity from others. Is it worth it?

4. How do you believe the problem should be treated? Include any medical or non-medical treatments you think would help you.

5. Have you ever been ill before at this same time of year?

6. Has this same problem/illness happened before?

7. Did your current problem/illness begin around the anniversary of some traumatic event like a death, divorce, car accident, hospitalization, etc.? This could even refer to an event many years past.

8. Do you want to rid yourself of this problem? Why?

9. Do you want to change yourself or someone else? Why?

10. What is this illness trying to teach you? Can you live with and learn from this problem? What could you learn?

11. Are you willing to resolve this conflict? If yes, What would it take? If no, Why not?

> *Serious illness doesn't bother me for long*
> *because I am too inhospitable a host.*
> —*Albert Schweitzer*

Self-Help Experience #8

21 Questions To Inventory Your Feelings

Purpose: To take an inventory of your common beliefs and attitudes about a variety of everyday experiences and events in order to uncover your feelings about them.

Many people go through life denying—not feeling—their feelings. Since dis-ease often results from ignored feelings acting on the body like underground invaders, it is important to allow these feelings to surface. Pay attention to your feelings as you read each question. Your "gut reactions" will be evidence of underground feelings that might affect you. It is possible to change the way you experience your body and the way your body reacts to you.

Ask yourself:

1. What do you expect from people?

2. Do you have a high, neutral or low opinion of most people?

3. Do most people take advantage of you or are they usually fair with you?

4. Are most people honest or dishonest?

5. How do you value your relationships?

6. Is work generally satisfying or frustrating?

7. How do you value your work?

8. Are you generally optimistic or pessimistic?

9. Do you expect life to serve you, or to do you in?

10. Do you feel you give more to others, or receive more from others?

11. Do you have enough money to satisfy your basic needs? Your desires?

12. Would more money make you happier?

13. Do you give generously?

14. Do you have integrity? Do you keep your word?

15. Do you generally like yourself?

16. Do you often feel "guilty"?

17. Is life often "too much to bear?"

18. Do you frequently desire revenge?

19. Do you often think... "What if?" "Why me?" "If only?"

If I have ever made any valuable discoveries, it has been owing more to patient observation than to any other reason.
—Isaac Newton

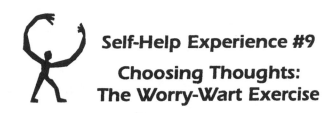

Self-Help Experience #9

Choosing Thoughts:
The Worry-Wart Exercise

Purpose: To practice being in charge of what you think about.

Instructions:

1. Choose to think some upsetting thoughts. Worry about something or someone. Think about something that makes you feel angry.

2. Stop thinking these thoughts. Tell yourself, "I release these upsetting thoughts and choose to think some happy thoughts." For example: Recall a happy incident. Think about someone you love. Imagine yourself winning a lot of money, or achieving a long-desired goal. Remember that God loves you.

3. Notice the difference in the way you feel when you are thinking these different types of thoughts.

4. Tell yourself, "I have the power to choose what I will think about." Do this whenever you find yourself beset by worries or negative thoughts.

The idea for this exercise came from Dennis Jaffee's *Healing From Within*, p. 124

Worry does not empty tomorrow of its sorrow; it
empties today of its strength.
—Corrie Ten Boom

I should have my head examined.

Get your hopes up.

Stick your neck out.

Chapter 5

Core Beliefs and Seedthoughts

There is a language connection between mind, body and emotions. Recent research has shown that much illness is self-created largely through this language. Words are often the trigger (catalyst) that lead to the symptoms of disease: you are what you think, feel, and say about yourself. *You are what you believe about you.*

Language is a tangible link between the emotional reality and thoughts of the mind and the physical reality of the body. Emotions can be expressed mentally and physically. The language of the mind is expressed in words and pictures through talking, writing, dreaming, mental imagining, visualizing, and fantasizing. The language of the body is expressed through both unpleasant and pleasant physical sensations like itching, sweating, rashes, pain, pressure, tears, laughter, smiles, orgasms, energy, and exuberance. Even a sneeze is part of the language connection, a loud clearly expressed response arising from a bodily need. Gross reactions to strong emotions include cold feet, sweaty palms, and the flush of excitement, among others.

Core beliefs and Seedthoughts

Core beliefs are the basic assumptions and ideas upon which your everyday thoughts and actions are based. These deeply held values lead to almost reflex-like knee jerk actions in response to circumstances and events in your life. You may not be conscious of your core beliefs and their accompanying seedthoughts, but your core belief system affects every part of your being—physical, mental, emotional, and spiritual. *Core beliefs can be altered by using consciously chosen seedthoughts.*

A "seedthought" is a significant catalyst for a physical or emotional response. A seedthought is a thought you think frequently that either emanates from, or creates, your core beliefs. Just as the apple core contains seeds that sprout into an apple tree, you have, at your core, beliefs which shape you.

Seedthoughts include the attitudes and emotions surrounding the thought. These seem to determine the potency of the seedthought, just as the soil around the seed determines the strength and vitality of the plant. A seedthought is an idea planted in the mind that grows into manifestation in the body. A seedthought can be health-promoting or, like a weed, choke out the life around it.

The body expresses in physical form both the positive and negative output of the mind. Thoughts and emotions stick to it, just as bits of salt stick to a pretzel, adding flavor and seasoning. Some seasoning enhances our experience of the pretzel. But too much salt often spoils the taste. So too, too much of certain types of thoughts and emotions can negatively affect the body.

Flakes As Feedback

For years before starting to write this book, I was involved in the presentation of new ideas such as women's liberation, holistic health, and spiritual healing. At one point, I was plagued by a persistent case of dandruff. Months of aggressive treatment failed to eliminate the ugly white flakes. I wondered if there was a language connection. I soon had the answer.

Frequently, while presenting new ideas, I would think: "They think I'm flaky," a perfect catalyst for dandruff. When I realized how clearly that thought was affecting me, I gasped. "They think I'm flaky" was indeed a thought that seemed to be the source of my dandruff, a perfect example of the creative role of language in the reactions and behaviors of my body. As I recognized the creative power of words, I began using the term "seedthought." What I had to do next was to verify that eliminating the seedthought would eliminate the physical condition of dandruff connected to it.

Recognizing the untruthfulness of "They think I'm flaky," I canceled the thought whenever it occurred to me. I realized that whether or not others saw me that way, the thought "I'm flaky" originated in my own mind and was solely my responsibility. Then I projected it onto others, creating a stubborn case of dandruff flakes in the process. I told myself the real truth, "I am not flaky! I am serious, thoughtful, fun, loving, and committed to new ideas. Many people who interact with me know that."

Within two weeks of my initial recognition of the flaky seedthought, and without further treatment, the dandruff disappeared. I had altered the belief underlying my seedthought when I acknowledged to myself that people did take me seriously. When I knew I wasn't flaky, I stopped flaking.

Since each person is unique, you might have different dandruff-related core beliefs; if you have dandruff, you might have a quite different seedthought. It is also possible to heal your unwanted condition *without* discovering a specific seedthought. Healing is self-induced when you recognize your responsibility and take appropriate physical, mental, and spiritual action.

Our Internal Chatter

The *Body* is a remarkable vehicle which allows us to feel physical sensations of pleasure and pain so we can learn from our experience.

The *Mind* speaks to us with words, pictures, or images (seedthoughts) which can translate into physical conditions in the body.

The *Spirit* is the life force within a body—the breath of life. We learn spiritual lessons related to love, compassion, and trust using mind and body. We are taught by feeling bodily experiences. Mind helps us to understand and create meaning, enabling us to grow as human (physical) and spiritual beings. *Spirit is the part of us that observes, understands, knows, grows, and loves.*

By observing our bodily reactions, we can discover seedthoughts and core beliefs which lurk beneath our conscious awareness. Seedthoughts like "I am flaky" are potent triggers that stimulate physical and emotional reactions in the body. Sometimes we recognize the seedthought after the fact. But at other times, we can catch ourselves in time for healthful re-programming or preventive medicine.

John Graham is a former NATO negotiator who now heads The Giraffe Project, an organization that acknowledges pioneers who "stick their necks out" by taking risks to improve the world. He told me, "I healed a persistent ache in my left foot by moving professionally in the right direction."[56] Just as the oyster turns the irritating grain of sand into a pearl, so too, humans can turn irritating experiences into experiences of personal growth.

Decoding Sensations

An intelligent approach to symptoms is to try and decode the meaning of the sensations in order to understand how to help your body. First check the physical basis of a sensation: Is it organic or is it functional? *Organic* means the sensation arises from the living tissue of the body—there is verifiable change or damage to a specific body part.

Functional pertains to dis-ease having no apparent physiological or structural cause. Something isn't working right and there is no known reason why. An example of this is *idiopathic* (unknown cause) *hypertension* (high blood pressure.) For hypertension there are several tests—for example, kidney X-rays—a doctor would use to try and determine the reason for the elevated blood pressure. If no physical cause is found, the disease is considered idiopathic. Helpful medical advice would then include a lifestyle re-assessment with suggestions for dietary changes, exercise, and tension-reducing activities. Exploring emotions is a useful part of this process. In any idiopathic disease, an exploration of the mental and emotional language connections can yield significant insights.

When I first wrote the above paragraph, I began looking for my own hypertension-related seedthoughts. I felt *pressured* to find some. "Grin and bear it," "Keep a stiff upper lip," and "Grit your teeth" are some I've come up with so far. And I'm still looking.

If you have a pain in the ribcage area, it might be caused by a cracked rib, or some other organic condition. If you've eliminated such possibilities, emotion or negative attitudes might be causing discomfort there. Your body usually reflects your underlying emotional condition. Tightness in the gut might relate to emotional tenseness as well as to problems from food, viruses, or other physical causes. Physical indigestion often results from the stress of emotional indigestion.

When decoding the meaning behind a symptom, *first rule out physical causes* and then look for emotional causes. Explore the emotional reasons for your dis-ease by searching for seedthoughts. If you often suffer from physical indigestion, examine your emotions to see if there is something in your life that "eats away at you" or "lies heavy in your gut." Perhaps you haven't "digested the meaning of an experience" or "assimilated an important life lesson." Maybe you are upset and "eating your heart out." Use your body's speech as a guide to the unconscious part of your mind. Then act on what you've discovered.

Many years ago, I had a severe rash. The itching and burning related to my anger, frustration, and impatience to get on with more important work—this book, for instance. But since there were other things I needed to do first, I had to learn patience. Recognizing the connection between my emotions and the allergic reactions enabled me to accept and release the underlying frustration, which helped my healing. Eventually I saw that I was actually working on the book all along and my ailments were part of the research process.

By witnessing sensations and symptoms in your body, your underlying pattern of beliefs becomes clear. Objective witnessing requires practice. It means observing, decoding, and understanding without negative self-judgment, blame, or punishment. If you are sick, you need to: *learn from the experience, forgive yourself and move on.*

Through the sensations in my body I often discover painful emotions. If I direct my energy and attention to a particular area, it usually begins to improve. Sometimes the problem first intensifies, just as using soap and water to clean a dirty shirt at first increases the mess, till dirt and soap wash out together.

Some days a pain in my gut reflects the hurt and unhappiness I feel or perhaps try to avoid feeling. Then I am literally *feeling* my feelings. Noticing my thoughts verifies the honesty of my body, as I discover what I am really thinking and feeling about something or someone.

Other days I almost purr like a kitten, reflecting a more positive state of mind. Since knowing myself and becoming a better person is my goal, I am grateful for the learning my body provides. An *attitude of gratitude* is important in the process of self-healing.

Chronic recurrences of a particular symptom may be the result of a well-defined mental blueprint. Different parts of the body speak to, as well as for, different people. Although there are typical patterns that many people exhibit, we each will have our own unique reactive language. For some who feel burdened, for instance, the back might act up. They have "too much to shoulder" or are "weighted down" with responsibility. For others, these same feelings might manifest as trouble with the weight-bearing parts—the joints of the leg, the knee, foot, or ankle.

Cliches As Emotional Expressions

Cliches often become seedthoughts which trigger dis-ease. These seedthoughts express emotion using words whose meaning relates directly to the symptoms evoked. For example, an expression most of us have used at one time or another is, "That _____ is a real pain in the neck, head, gut, or ass." (You fill in the blank.) We are generally expressing our feelings about some particular thing or situation. But saying "that is a real pain in the whatever" can actually trigger a painful stiff neck, an upset stomach, or a real headache. Your spoken words *may* match a particular symptom exactly, triggering that symptom as a sensation (dis-ease) in your body.

The process also works in reverse. You may begin using those expressions after you first physically feel something amiss. For example, if you have real physical distress from a stiff neck or an upset stomach, you may want to talk about how you feel. So saying "that was a pain in the neck" or "that gave me an upset stomach" is true; you do already have a sore neck or an upset stomach. The seedthought stimulating your physical distress *is then reinforced by the distress as you feel it*, strengthening your original symptom-triggering thought. Your *belief* in whatever that _____ is that gives you such distress is stored in your unconscious mind. Then just thinking the seedthought "that _____ will give me whatever" can trigger the physical distress. But discovery of the seedthought can break the disease cycle.

"My nerves are raw" is another statement many people use to express some kind of emotional upset. But that seedthought too can be stored in the mind, and later "solidified" in the body, resulting in pain and inflammation. Here too, the words used match the actual symptoms present in many diseases, among them the painful condition called arthritis. The nerves can be raw and painful in the body of an arthritis sufferer. Your body often takes your words quite literally and creates what you've spoken of.

In order to move from being a victim to a victor, it is necessary to mentally recognize and accept your feelings and then eliminate any negative verbal expressions. Like Charlie Brown, don't keep asking, "Why's everybody always pickin' on me?" Instead be like Annie who sings, "the sun will come out tomorrow..."

Discovering Your Seedthoughts

A common seedthought for some people is a name. The mere mention of someone against whom we harbor ill feelings can cause untold distress and wreak havoc on one's body. Mentioning the name of someone we love deeply can bring feelings of joy, love and pleasure, or fear of loss. The loss of a loved one can result in pain and despair when remembering the beloved; even if the relationship ended because you wanted to end it, the name can retain the power to evoke a physical or emotional reaction.

Any thought can stimulate us. However, we each have basic seedthoughts which can stimulate predictable reactions whenever we think that thought. An example of this occurs in people prone to the panic of acute anxiety. Just thinking they are on the verge of anxiety can lead them to the sensations of anxiety. Their bodymind has learned that sweating, shaking, tightening muscles and nausea are some of the sensations that accompany anxiety and it will begin to produce those symptoms in the presence of the seedthought "I am having an anxiety attack."

An individual afraid of stuttering when speaking is more likely to stutter. Neurology and psychiatry professor Viktor Frankl calls this "anticipatory anxiety."[57] Frankl wrote of the irony that *fear makes come true what one is afraid of and what one forcibly wishes for often brings the opposite result.* "The more a man tries to demonstrate his sexual potency or a woman her ability to experience orgasm, the less they are able to succeed."[58] A fearful expectation often leads right to the undesirable result; wanting something so much, yet believing it won't happen, can block its happening.

Which Comes First, Chicken or Egg?

Notice how you explain your physical sensations. You may tell yourself you are sick or you may tell yourself you are well. Sometimes you ignore physical sensations, but *subconsciously, every thought tells your body how to react.* Each thought promotes health or illness. The internal dialogue goes on in drumbeat time whether you hear it or not. Once an idea has gained a foothold in your physical world, other thoughts, words and images may affect its existence. Still, a core belief can be so powerful that contrary evidence disproving that belief might be ignored.

Words are not the sole cause of dis-ease. But, they certainly are a link in a chain of causative factors that includes among others environment, lifestyle, and heredity. Words create the climate that allows disease to flourish. Language affects the quality of life.

There is no final, definitive evidence yet that the words you speak actually cause disease or whether they simply reflect what is already present. There appears to be some truth in both these points of view. *At times, we develop physical disease just to allow us to experience our thoughts and emotions, so that we can recognize and change them.* The language of the body/mind connection works in two ways:

• Sometimes your emotions become physical problems;

• Sometimes your physical problems lead you to recognize your emotions.

We don't always know which comes first, the chicken or the egg, the thought or the emotion, the disease or the feelings. And perhaps people do recognize the language of their body/mind connection whenever they use that common old saying, "I should have my head examined."

Self-Help Experience #10

Self-Awareness

Purpose: To expand your ability to recognize your seedthoughts and core beliefs; to learn how your memories affect you; to recognize thoughts on which you may have patterned your life.

Instructions:

1. *Have a paper and pen handy so that you can write down your discoveries at the end of this exercise.* Read through all the instructions, or read all the instructions onto a tape. Once you are comfortably settled, close your eyes for a few moments to block out any external stimuli. This exercise works with eyes opened or closed. But, if you have trouble recognizing your feelings, then closing your eyes will improve your results.

2. *Notice how you are feeling right now.* Observe your thoughts, feelings and any physical sensations. Describe to yourself the way different parts of your body feel. Do you have uncomfortable physical sensations? What is your emotional state? Are you happy, sad, angry, bored, excited, curious, interested, or something else? As you follow the rest of these instructions, notice any changes.

3. *Think about some thing, incident, or person that made you angry.* Become aware of all the details of the scene: who was there, what they were wearing, the colors around you, where you were, the expressions on people's faces, and so on. Really remember what anger was like and describe your physical sensations as you think about your anger. Notice if you can re-experience the anger in your mind, to see how it feels physically and emotionally.

See if your sensations change as you allow yourself to remember and observe your experience. Sometimes an emotion like anger will disappear after a few moments and be replaced by another emotion, perhaps sadness, or even compassion.

(continued) next page

4. *Recall a time when you were happy.* Recall in detail what went on at that time. Really remember what being happy was like and describe your physical sensations as you think about being happy. Notice if you can re-experience that time in your mind, to see how it feels physically and emotionally.

5. *Think of the name of someone you love.* How does that name, and the image of that person, make you feel? Describe your physical sensations as you think about your loved one.

6. *Now remember someone you once loved, but who is no longer in your life.* See how that memory makes you feel. Describe your physical sensations as you think about this person.

Observe your physical sensations, thoughts, and feelings as you examine any situation in your life that upsets you. Use this process to release emotion whenever you need to be clear-headed. This exercise is especially helpful when you are problem-solving or prior to major lifestyle changes such as a new job, a new home, marriage or divorce, and so on.

When you become aware of how your memories and underlying beliefs are affecting you right now, you will be motivated to make the changes that will improve your life. The rest of this book and many of the exercises to come will help you to make those changes that mend the mind and heal the body. There are many techniques for you to use to help you to "think yourself healthy." But, becoming aware by observing yourself living your life is effective even by itself.

Assure a quality tomorrow by leaving sad yesterdays far behind.
—Author Unknown

Self-Help Experience #11

Changing Upsetting Thoughts

Purpose: To give you practice in changing your mind to control the effects of your emotions. Being upset will simply add more power and energy to a negative thought, thus reinforcing it. You can abort an anxiety attack with this harmonizing technique.

Instructions:

1. *Release a negative thought by saying a particular word or phrase, like "cancel," "God forbid," or "delete."* Consider your brain as operating like a computer. You are simply giving it the command to abort whatever is going on right now. For example, your internal dialogue might go like this: "This project is a headache. Cancel, cancel."

After you cancel, replace the negative thought with a positive one of your choosing. For example: "This project is very challenging." From this perspective, you will be reprogramming your mind in a more positive way.

2. *Visualize (imagine) yourself taking an eraser and erasing the negative thought.* Then consciously create a positive image to replace the erased thought. For example, first visualize your previous negative image of a specific project. In your mind's eye, see the image being rubbed away by your mental eraser. In the place of the previous image, picture an image of what the successfully completed project would look like. You might then see yourself celebrating the successful completion of your challenging project.

I sometimes had trouble writing when my mind created thoughts of failure, leading me to fear and frustration. After noting those feelings, I'd release the stimulus thoughts and change my mind. I spent many happy moments imagining this manuscript done, finding an agent, and finally being published.

I *saw* the completed book. I *felt* my happiness. I imagined myself on TV, making a major speech somewhere or signing autographs in bookstores. I frequently imagined my book on a best-seller list. Pretending like this often motivated me to write when I felt like doing something else.

A pessimist is one who makes difficulties of his opportunities, and an optimist is one who makes opportunities of his difficulties.
—Harry Truman

That breaks my heart.

I'm itching to get on with it.

My head isn't screwed on straight.

Chapter 6

Emotion and Your Body's Language

I discovered the true power of seedthoughts by observing and experiencing my body and then noticing what I was thinking and saying. For example, I used to say, *"I don't have my head on straight,"* referring to my emotional life. I paid no attention then to the literal meaning of my words. I used those words as a feeble excuse for some imperfection in my behavior. I thought this was a good idea, but this belittling myself, putting myself down, was really a self-defeating habit.

Then, one day in 1976, I tripped while walking in the woods. My neck and the muscles holding my spine in place felt sore. Being cautious, I went to a chiropractor for treatment. I thought I would be fine. A week later, while walking in New York City, I felt something in my neck move, heard a crunching noise, and experienced intense fear.

Over the next few days I noticed my neck sloping off at an angle. To counterbalance the angle of my neck, the weight of my head went towards the opposite direction. *"My head is not on straight"* had become an accurate statement about my body. I became aware of the language connection between my body and my crooked neck when I finally noticed how frequently I talked about not being straight. I don't talk that way anymore. Which came first, the injury or the statement? I honestly don't remember.

Dr. Robert Marshall, a chiropractor, provides a similar example of how beliefs can affect the body. He said:

"A new patient came to me for an adjustment. Her body was very misaligned. One shoulder was considerably higher than the other. She looked almost crooked. I suggested that she go home and look at herself in the mirror.

"When she returned for her next visit, she shared her astonishment at really looking at her body and seeing for the first time how crookedly she presented herself to the world. Looking in the mirror she discovered a seedthought taught to her in childhood: *'Don't be straight with people.'* She saw those words clearly reflected in her crooked body. This patient told me that she had considerable difficulty in being with people. She never was straight with them, even though she wanted to be. Her family taught her dishonesty by telling her not to be up front with people. 'Keep your feelings to yourself. Don't show your hand. Never be straight with people.' Consequently, facing people straight and looking them in the eye was difficult. And her body was very crooked."[59]

Emotional Connections to the Past

During my childhood my mother repeated over and over, *"If you don't have something nice to say, don't say it."* As a result, I was prone to hide certain "not nice" feelings from others, turning them inward upon myself. I too was taught not to be straight with people, and I too have a body that isn't straight.

Hiding feelings and storing them in my body required a great deal of energy, resulting in excess stress and muscle tension. Resentment builds up quickly. Sometimes I'd explode and dump anger on those I love. Unexpressed feelings of sadness might send me on a crying jag unconnected to a specific event.

Now I can choose to release these feelings by being more straight with people from the beginning. Being straight with people was a major issue in my life. I don't mean to criticize my mother for teaching me to speak kindly. On the contrary, I appreciate the fact that she planted such words in my heart. But, I really don't have to hide my feelings. I can express them in a way that is helpful to others. Expressing anger, sadness or disappointment can be useful feedback to the recipient, especially if tempered with love.

Writer Tony Schwartz describes the following experience related to chronic stress:

"Three years ago, I was suffering from chronic back pain despite two years of visits to every imaginable kind of specialist. Finally I went to see a doctor named John Sarno, at NYU's Rusk Institute, who believes that virtually all back pain is due not to structural causes but to stress. Sarno treats back pain by giving a series of lectures on the physiology and psychology of tension. He teaches the power of the mind over the body. Period. My pain went away within several weeks and has never returned. I have since sent more than forty back-pain sufferers to Sarno, including at least a half-dozen with herniated disks. All but one of the forty were pain-free within a matter of weeks."[60]

Memories also trigger bodily sensations. Memory, in fact, is often attached to emotion. We tend to remember those experiences that initially elicited a strong emotional reaction in us. Names of people important to us from the past and in the present can become seedthoughts. The name can evoke a physical response and emotional reaction because it symbolizes feelings related to love or loss of love, hate, anger or even fear. We can revisit a relationship years later and alter past negative connections.

Several years ago I saw a man with whom I had once shared a very emotional year. I was excited and nervous about seeing him again. Our friendship was deep, perhaps more so because we weren't lovers. Although I was relieved when the relationship ended, the pain at the end was strong. The mere thought of him or hearing his name triggered a physical reaction in me. I felt like I was being punched from within, with a tightness in my gut, pressure and heat in my chest, and a heart that would start racing. His name and my image of him had become a seedthought and my body showed me, back then, that I missed him.

For a whole year after we stopped meeting, I processed and released my emotions associated with that relationship. I was very unhappy, mourning the pain of other lost loves as I experienced long-suppressed emotions. It is common for unexpressed grief to be stored in the body and triggered by fresh loss. My release of grief was definitely health-producing.

I thought I was completely healed of the hurt and no longer missed him, but I was uncertain of my subconscious reaction to being with him. After seeing him again I felt fine, but still I wondered if I was fooling myself, suppressing my emotions, still missing him. A dream symbolically showed me I was really okay. In my dream we sat in a car, preparing to go to a movie. We acknowledged our love for each other. Then I kissed him goodbye, saying, "I choose to be somewhere else—not with you." Then I left the car. This dream confirmed that I am okay whether I see him or not.

The effect of grief on the body has long been reported in the medical literature. James Lynch, a doctor specializing in psychosomatic medicine, writing in *The Broken Heart,* makes a strong case for the effects of grief and separation on the human heart. He notes that "Drs. Kraus and Lillienfeld, in 1959, using data published by the National Office of Vital Statistics, were among the first to call attention to the abrupt rise in mortality among widows and widowers, especially in the young widowed group."[61] People do express their grief in their bodies and they can and do die of "broken hearts."

Libby, a nurse, wrote via e-mail:

"After the premature death of our rabbi, a close friend, from a sudden and massive heart attack, our own hearts were stricken with grief and pain. I myself suffered angina and a very mild heart attack. I always knew that people could die from grief—I saw that happen to my own parents—and now I have had a warning that it could happen to me.

"My parents both died of heart failure on the same day at the same time; they always told us they were 'soul-mates.' They died on the birthday of my brother Carl who had preceded them in death from cancer; they never got over losing Carl who was the 'baby' of the family, and often said they were too 'heart-broken' to go on with life after that. The rest of us were sad, but not surprised that they went out together from heart-failure.

"Anyhow, I've had my cardiac warning; now it's up to me to focus on positive change in my own life. Fortunately, I am very blessed with the love and support of my wonderful husband!"[62]

Divorce and separation likewise produce immunological changes according to researchers Kiecolt and Glaser. In one study, they found that those women who had been separated one year or less had poorer immune function than a well-matched control group of married women. It was also reported that people with fewer close relationships have higher rates of disease and death.[63] What happens in one's interpersonal relationships does have health consequences.

You Are the Meaning Maker

Emotions and your overall sense of illness or well-being are felt and expressed in your body. Your general feeling of illness or wellness is a purely subjective evaluation which you make for yourself. Often it relates to your general emotional state. You can physically feel, as well as speak of or act out, the emotions of happiness, joy, anger, sadness, or grief. You feel happiness when you laugh or smile. Anger is felt as muscle tension, a churning in the gut, or even a rise in body temperature. Tears give physical expression to sadness, joy, or grief.

You, as the one who says what something means, can discover the *why* of each physical sensation. Pay attention to your body and think about what a feeling means. Body conditions reflect emotional attitudes. So, people with severe illness such as heart disease, cancer, arthritis, or even AIDS, should be treated for underlying emotional distress. Even if their seedthoughts remain a mystery, healing will still be facilitated.

Seedthoughts often interconnect, forming a pattern for the body. More than one set of thoughts may be responsible for triggering the form, shape, and condition of your body. Similarly, a series of interconnected beliefs can affect your emotions. Eliminating any one seedthought can have the effect of toppling the whole dis-easing structure. But more extensive work might be necessary in order to change the negative blueprint which you have been using to create your physical and emotional reality.

Citing innumerable studies and case histories in *SUPER IMMUNITY: Master Your Emotions and Improve Your Health*, Paul Pearsall, Ph.D. , demonstrates the roles of mind and emotion in all disease. He investigates the crucial link between your state of mind and your health, and the need to allow healing to occur by knowing, loving, and accepting yourself. Pearsall writes:

"Epidemiology, the study of large numbers of people and emerging patterns of disease, also points to the importance of the psychosomatic relationship. In 1976, Dr. C.B. Thomas published results of a study of medical students who were followed for thirty years. She found that profiles of psychological tests were predictive of such sicknesses as cancer, heart disease and high blood pressure. Dr. George Valiant conducted a similar study published in 1974 and 1977. In his study, a large population of Harvard students was followed for thirty years, and the relationship between emotional maturity and disease vulnerability was clearly shown."[64]

There is mounting scientific evidence and increased understanding of a direct physical mechanism uniting the brain, the mind, the emotions and the immune system. Messenger molecules called neuropeptides, transmitted through virtually all the body fluids (blood, lymph, etc.) seem to link the immune, endocrine, and central nervous systems.

A Rash Experience: Actions & Antidotes

Examining my physical sensations, I often recognize emotions I was unconscious of feeling. Frequently, I discover many seedthoughts that are interconnected—my own negative blueprint. For instance, several language connections became apparent to me at a time when I was being "attacked" by body rashes. Three times in six weeks, I broke out in a horrendous rash all over my body. I itched! I burned! The rashes seemed to result from food allergies. But equally, the rashes were messages resulting from deeply felt, but unrecognized emotions.

My doctor reassured me that the condition was not a serious disease. It looked and felt worse than it actually was. After a while I was able to see the experience as an opportunity to learn about myself and transform my relationship to the part of me that is my body. "Being itchy" related to being impatient. "Burning up" expressed my unacknowledged anger in a physical way. I felt ugly and unclean.

"Hexaba" was a name I used then to refer to the ugly, bad part of me—the seething network of unexpressed negative emotions and seedthoughts. She was in my unconscious, screaming to get out, to be accepted and loved. She expressed herself through my body, and conceptualizing and naming her was my attempt to make a painful life-experience meaningful.

I kept saying how ugly the rash was, but I didn't hide. Wearing makeup was out of the question. My skin was too sensitive, my lips cracked and burned. I often asked my family to look at the rash: "How does it look? Is it improving or getting worse?" There was a dichotomy between believing I looked ugly and wanting everyone to see me. I attended a wedding and had my picture taken in order to remember that time. Soon the ugliness I felt inside was leaving. My skin was a mirror of what was going on inside me. I was learning, through the reflection provided by my skin and the loving concern of friends and family, to love, accept, and forgive myself. It wasn't the first, nor the last, time that my body was my teacher.

I recognized that I was responsible for this rash, perhaps because of erratic and overindulgent food habits, as well as embedded patterns of self-hate. Discovering the food connection helped me heal the rash and the physical behaviors stemming from my underlying emotional pattern. My body's suffering made me more aware of certain problem areas and provided me with an incentive for deeper self-examination, change, and transformation.

As I recognized my seedthoughts, I created mental antidotes to change my unhealthy core beliefs and alter my emotional reactions. I would frequently repeat positive affirmations to myself in order to counteract the harmful core beliefs. I also played video games in my mind, visualizing "Pacmen" as robotic vacuum cleaners, or even miniature doctors wearing white-coats, coursing through my body; clearing out foreign invaders; gobbling up germs, allergens, tumors, and fats. Soon afterward, the rashes on my body disappeared and I lost fifteen pounds. These mental processes were used in conjunction with physical techniques such as an altered diet, exercising, and herbal remedies. The seedthoughts and core beliefs I discovered—and their antidotes—included:

Seedthought and Symptom: I am itching.

> **Core Belief:** I felt emotionally at odds with myself. I was itching to move on to the next cycle in my life, to begin writing this book.

> **Mental Antidote:** I am moving as fast as I really want to. I am more patient each day.

Seedthought and Symptom: I am burning up. The rash was so red hot it burned my skin.

> **Core Belief:** Burning up was indicative to me of my stored anger burning me as it was released through my skin.

> **Mental Antidote:** I transform the warmth within to love and peace. I am cool and at ease.

Seedthought and Symptom: I am ugly. The rash was gross looking.

> **Core Belief:** I felt as if poison was coming out of me both physically and spiritually; the poison of self-hate and anger.

> **Mental Antidote:** I am beautiful and purifying my soul.

During my rash experience I checked with an internist and a dermatologist to rule out serious organic disease. There was no specific medical treatment but the dermatologist reassured me that this condition wasn't as serious as it appeared, just ugly and uncomfortable. He said,"This too shall pass," a reassuring affirmation. Who is to say which of the things I did was most responsible for my healing? The one thing I am sure of is that I learned a lot about myself and grew emotionally from this experience.

The skin is an easily viewed mirror of our unconscious state. It can be restored to health by changing our thinking. Pearsall writes of a boy with a so-called incurable skin condition called *congenital ichthyosiform erythrodermia*, which results in hardening and blackening of the skin. He writes, "All major dermatology textbooks report no known cure for this terrible disease. Hypnotist Dr. Mason saw the boy and offered mental imagery suggestions to relax him and to help him learn to see his skin as becoming normal. Within ten days the skin had returned to normal. Dr. Mason's results, published in the *British Medical Journal*, were later verified by three other medical researchers." Other physicians later obtained positive results in improving other skin disorders. Concludes Pearsall, "We now know that 'T-cell-mediated skin response' relates to our emotions and beliefs, that the skin reacts intensely to our feelings."[65]

Jack, a former student of mine, often talked angrily as if he was "itching to clobber someone." All the while he was scratching the white scaly patches on his arms. In many ways a gentle soul who would never knowingly hurt anyone, Jack's anger was nevertheless intense. Unwilling to face himself as the true source of this anger, Jack's skin provided an outlet for his emotions. With no place to go, it "oozed out of his body," leading to the itchy rash of psoriasis.

Mind Over Matter

Dr. Barbara Brown[66] used her background in brain and behavior research in her book *Supermind: The Ultimate Energy*. But her personal experience was useful too. After being told that she required a tonsillectomy, she spent time preparing her emotions before surgery. She wrote: "From time to time I would silently tell myself that the operation would be easy, cause no pain, and that there would be no problems." The operation, done without anesthetic, went well, she "felt no pain, didn't bleed and had absolutely no recovery problems. Mind over matter. This hidden capacity of mind to control the vital functions of the body has been useful to me at other times, although I confess I do not know what happens in the mind to accomplish such remarkable effects. I do know that I *will* it...."

Another time Brown nearly amputated her thumb in a household accident. After a surgeon sewed up the damage, she returned home, without stopping for pain pills. Again using the power of her mind, she repeatedly told herself that she would feel no pain. Because the surgeon had warned her that the thumb would be numb and disfigured, she added the command for the thumb to heal whole again, without scars. Between her mental suggestions and a few stiff drinks, she kept the pain at bay. "The thumb healed quickly, with only a faint line as reminder."

I have come to know myself better by observing my thoughts, experiencing my feelings, and seeing the effect of each on my body. In the long run, this self-awareness enables me to live a happier, more productive life. It has also become abundantly clear that words are mental things which we embody with meaning. We can unmask our body and discover the meaning it has. Just as we can uncover seedthoughts to find the patterns leading to dis-ease in our body, we can choose seedthoughts to create newer, healthier patterns to live by. *If our words and thoughts can make us ill, they can also make us well.*

Self-Help Experience #12

Mirror Feedback

Purpose: To gather information about you by really looking at your body; to provide practice in observing yourself and seeing yourself as you look to others. This experience is strictly to gather information. This enhanced self-awareness often leads to healing without doing anything.

Instructions:

1. *Stand naked in front of a full length mirror.* Take several deep breaths to relax your body. Observe the way your body looks, without trying to make it look better. Is it straight? Is one shoulder higher than the other? Do you slouch?

The mirror facilitates self-observance because some people never look at themselves as they really are. They will suck in their tummy, or stand tall or smile to make themselves look better.

2. *Notice any thoughts you have while you are looking at your body.* If you are judging your body, notice how the judgments make you feel.

3. *Thank your body for supporting you throughout your life* after you have finished observing yourself. Do this out loud. For example, "I give thanks for my body—the vehicle through which I experience my life."

Do what you can with what you have, with where you are.
—Theodore Roosevelt

Self-Help Experience #13

Names As Seedthoughts

Purpose: To realize the power of memories.

Instructions:

1. Close your eyes. Relax. Repeat the name of someone who has been very important in your life. The image of that person, or the thought of that name, probably evokes powerful emotions within—perhaps joy, or sadness, or even anger. Your body is smart; it knows the physical sensations to produce for each emotion or memory.

2. Use your own name as a positive seedthought. Look in the mirror and tell yourself, "I love and appreciate you (say your name). Add a reason. For example, I might say, "I love and appreciate you, Barbara, because you are willing to dredge up your unconscious emotions and write about them to help others." The more reasons you can come up with the better. Do this as a daily exercise when you brush your teeth.

Don't be too timid and squeamish about your
actions. All life is an experiment. The more
experiments you make the better.
—Ralph Waldo Emerson

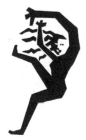

Something is eating away at me.

Eat your heart out.

A bitter pill to swallow.

Chapter 7

The Body As Emotional Barometer

At one time I believed I had a "stomach like a rock," that I could digest anything without stomach upset. The positive side of the seedthought "I have a stomach like a rock" comes from the notion that a strong stomach can "take it," implying also a strong person who can "take it." This belief reflected what I thought was my healthy digestive system. Then, at age 34, gallstones were found. The accepted treatment at the time was the removal of the gallbladder and I duly underwent that operation. I then began to notice food-related problems and paid more attention to what I ate.

Years later, during a meditation I recognized the language connection between the seedthought "stomach like a rock" and some digestive difficulties. Rocks are actually heavy and indigestible. Carrying rocks around is a burden. Early on, the seedthought helped me to believe I was invulnerable to so-called unhealthy eating habits. But actually, I needed to be careful about the food I ingested physically and the thoughts I ingested emotionally. When I ate foolishly and had fearful thoughts, I developed digestive problems. When I released negativity and worry, my digestive difficulties eased. This release is vital. One Eastern mystic dramatized it with the words, "If you are happy enough, you can digest rocks." My body has been an excellent vehicle for learning about the language connection.

Eating Right to Stay Fit

My involvement in holistic healing led me to work on improving my body through better nutrition. For years I followed a vegetarian health food diet, not worrying much about my digestion. By studying with different teachers, I learned many alternative approaches to eating. Among the eating plans I tried then were the Grafs' low stress system, Macrobiotics, Natural Hygiene, the Pritikin diet, and a raw food and vegetable juice diet. Some things were common to all—mostly vegetarian and no sugar—but there were major differences.

I tried each new eating plan believing it would improve my health. In my quest for better health, I was often very confused about what to eat. I knew people who had successfully used each one of these eating plans. My ever-improving well-being pleased me. I even lost weight easily. But then, after succumbing to thoughts like "This is boring, too rigid, or too difficult to maintain," I would fall back to eating almost anything. As I became aware of the rules of these different eating plans, I often thought: "Am I damaging my health by the food I am eating?" The dialogue in my head was characterized by fear and confusion. Which eating plan was I to follow? Which rules should I keep, and which should I break?

Fear acts as a magnet for negative experiences. Focusing too much attention on avoiding something really puts energy into what you don't want. As part of the physical universe we are all subject to the Law of Gravity—"what goes up must come down." So too, we are all subject to the principle of consciousness called the Law of Attraction—"what you think about comes about." Fear, based on negative core beliefs, creates a negative expectation that can become a self-fulfilling prophecy. I knew this intellectually.

No matter how good the food was, my mental nourishment was rich in anxiety. Since I couldn't follow every one of these mutually incompatible diets, what if I was choosing the wrong one? I had too much conflicting information, so I had to make choices. The fear of doing the wrong thing attended any course I chose. It seems that I had unknowingly programmed myself for digestive problems, no matter what I ate.

One day, at a workshop I heard myself say, "Something is eating away at me." I wasn't talking about food. But I soon recognized the food-related connection and meaning of my seedthought, "Something is eating away at me." This insight triggered the start of releasing my food fears, my impatience, and my digestive upsets.

All my digestive system beliefs were intertwined. Once I had found the key seedthoughts behind them, they began to unravel, taking many forms. I had been afraid of food and confused about an appropriate nutritional eating plan for myself. I had past programming related to every type of food I ate—it might be too fatty, or bad for circulation, or hard to digest when eaten in combination with certain other foods, like no meat with potatoes. That diet emphasized food combining. I seemed to be allergic to some foods. I was concerned about preservatives, or that the food was dead and lacking in enzymes. When eating out, I'd worry about improper handling and food spoilage.

There were days when everything I ate triggered some fear. In spite of this, I still loved to eat, but my worrisome thoughts contributed to heightened stress and reduced my sense of well-being. I realized that no matter how good my life got, no matter how peaceful the world became, I would not be at peace until I eliminated my food-related fears. I resolved to let go of fearful food-related thoughts, to eat food, and think thoughts that helped me.

I made a major shift of context as *I pictured my past patterns and unhealthy beliefs being eaten away.* I took that recurrent, unhelpful seedthought, "Something is eating away at me", and turned it against my negative beliefs. In this way, a once-negative thought became a vehicle for my own transformation. Now I eat what I want, whenever I want, in response to more health-promoting seedthoughts.

The Body Speaks Its Mind

The body is a barometer for emotions. You may be unconscious of negativity or upset, but discomfort in your body can point out your emotional distress. Memories often trigger the desire to eat. Many people eat more than necessary when under stress. Alice Katz, psychotherapist and author of *Conquering Compulsive Eating and Eating Without Guilt*, said:

"We use food inappropriately to feed an emotion like loneliness. But loneliness requires people for true comfort. Eating is a way we both express and cover up emotion. What we eat, when we eat and why we eat can be related to memories and unconscious beliefs.

"One overweight woman client loved pasta. She remembered going to a buffet with her favorite uncle. She took a large plateful of food and then was praised by her family when she went to get more pasta. Another client recalled not being allowed to have candy as a child. Candy was 'forbidden fruit.' For spite, when she got older, she ate candy in great quantities. Eating was her act of defiance: an inappropriate behavior that hurt her as much as anyone."[67]

My sister Arlene often said, "I ate my way through Barbara's brain surgery." She used food to drown her fearful feelings. In time she stopped *using food as a cover-up.* When my sister found more appropriate ways to express her emotions, the excess weight appeared to melt off her. Arlene is a role model who reminds us that it is possible to break the habit of swallowing feelings.

A research study by Marvin Acklin and Gene Alexander[68] described in *Brain/Mind Bulletin* found a clear association between inability to express emotion and a variety of illnesses from gastrointestinal disorders to dermatitis, migraines, and low back pain. For example:

Jean, a homemaker's assistant, once had a ghastly case of twenty-four-hour stomach flu that actually lasted days longer. At the end, she recognized how her sensitivity to stressful feelings had made her more vulnerable to this awful physical upset. She said "I trapped myself in a job with an employer I dislike." By its physical reactions, her body showed Jean how unhappy she was. As soon as she was well enough to work, she changed jobs.

Lillian, a writer, talked about the intestinal pain she suffered during divorce proceedings. She said "My gut feeling was that there was nothing physically wrong. Still I was in lots of pain. Tests showed I was physically okay. Eventually I realized that I simply *'couldn't stomach'* what was going on in this divorce."

Jack, an engineer and a self-improvement junkie, often asked me for self-help advice. Something seemed to be "eating away at him"—he was never satisfied. He spoke of his " gut-level negative programming," which he had to get rid of. Doctors eventually discovered that Jack had a long-standing case of intestinal parasites.

Bernie Siegel, M.D., in *Love, Medicine and Miracles* wrote about a comment from one of his patients after emergency surgery to remove several feet of dead intestine. Siegel really listened to his patients so they often shared their true feelings with him. This patient, a Jungian therapist, told Siegel, "I'm glad you're my surgeon, I've been undergoing teaching analysis. I couldn't handle all the shit that was coming up, or digest the crap in my life."[69]

Distressing or negative feelings often arise after we commit ourselves to something that really stretches our abilities. For fifteen years, Henry, a student of mine, was general manager of Jim's profitable wholesale business. When Jim retired, Henry purchased the business using borrowed capital. For the next ten years, Henry struggled to repay the loan and grow the business, working long, hard hours. Managing a business that he owned really stretched his abilities. Henry often said, "Thoughts like, 'Why did I ever buy this business?' keep intruding on my mind. Pressure to repay the loans and keep the business viable don't give me much time or energy for myself. I often feel isolated;

there's no one to share this burden. I feel a hunger and to satisfy it, I eat too much and gain weight."

During his limited free time Henry often complained of headaches and other vague discomforts. His feelings of inadequacy, fear of failure, and general discomfort at being the boss were struggling to be acknowledged. Eventually Henry got the message from his body. He realized that his physical discomforts were telling him to change his attitudes and lifestyle. He alleviated the stress with more rest, relaxation and exercise, and less food. During counseling he realized that he had many choices. He told me, "I could close down the business, or hire someone else to run it, or even sell it. Work was meant to enhance my life, not replace it."

Since Henry was still committed to his business, he hired more people to assist him—a step he had been reluctant to take. He said: "I blew it and now I am going to resurrect it." After getting in touch with the fear and self-doubt that had impeded his ability to make wise choices, he ran the business with renewed awareness. Clearing up the emotional stress released the pain, helping his body to feel better. Feeling better helped him to think more clearly. Henry had digested his past experiences, assimilated information which motivated him to eliminate negative thoughts and make many positive changes. Henry recently said, "In the past, I lacked confidence in my abilities. But now, I know I have what it takes to get the job done. I am good at, and enjoy being, a problem solver." Henry's seedthoughts are now self-enhancing not self-defeating.

Dr. Larry Novik, a primary care specialist in Bridgeport, Connecticut, speaking on a panel of medical professionals, talked about a patient who came to see him because, that day, she began having trouble talking. Dr. Novik said:

"It looked like her tongue was darting uncontrollably in and out of her mouth, perhaps a result of some unexplained muscle spasm. In taking her history, I found out that that morning, an unexpected job workload was unfairly placed on her. Although she was overwhelmed by the work load, she was unable to say anything.

"I led her in a relaxation exercise during which the muscles would release and then go right back into spasm. Finally I said to her 'You must be really angry at the way they treated you at work today.' She began to cry and immediately the spasm stopped and the problem was resolved.

"This case showed me how incredibly powerful our emotions are. We express ourselves through our body. Emotions can dictate what will happen to our bodies. Then, I realized that by experiencing and giving voice to the original emotion, such as when the patient began to cry, the bodily symptoms disappear. I saw that we can create a diseased or a healthy body by what we are feeling, thinking and saying or not saying.

"Emotions play a pivotal role in disease, and we as physicians need to pay attention to that part of our patients. It's not always that fast and easy to eliminate a painful symptom during an office visit, but I always keep in my mind that my patients thoughts and feelings might be making them sick."[70]

Pow! That Emotion Just Zapped You

A common core belief is that our lives would be great if we could control the external circumstances. That sounds right to many people and yet evidence abounds to the contrary. The true quality of our lives comes from our internal response.

For example: one man goes bankrupt and commits suicide, and another learns from the experience and goes on to be successful. One woman gets cancer and bemoans her fate; another uses the experience to make deep inner changes, emerging happier and more peaceful. Some people get yelled at and scream back verbal abuse. Others listen with understanding and compassion, adding peace to a troubled environment. One driver lets you cut in line in front of him, another honks his horn and gives you the finger.

These responses come from different inner attitudes, and surely the felt experience of each is different. *Each of us determines the quality of our lives through the core beliefs that influence our behavior.*

To understand how emotions affect us, it is helpful to understand something about the basic nature of emotion. Emotions are real—a strong surge of feeling! These feelings are automatic reactions that reflect our past experiences. Emotions are the primal (original, archetypal, fundamental) instinctive parts of our being. Therapist Julia Bondi, author of *Lovelight: Un-*

veiling the Mysteries of Sex and Romance believes that instinctive emotional reactions to situations can help us recognize unconscious core beliefs. She explained it this way:

"We have evolved beyond being only instinctual-reactive emotional creatures. We now have the power of thought—a gift from God—to use to harness the energy of our emotions. Emotions as responses are always there, ready to be felt. Experience stimulates them. Thinking about things does too! We react emotionally and the explanation we give ourselves to express and cope with what we instinctively feel, can develop into an unconscious belief. In a sense, we feel the emotion and then attempt to explain away any hurt.

Because emotions are primal or instinctive, the mind and thought is our way of both getting in touch with them and also directing them appropriately. Reacting off of emotions, without thinking things through, often leads us to say or do things that we'll later regret. Conscious thought helps us deal with our emotions constructively, as long as we don't use our thoughts to judge or deny them. Right thinking allows us to change our inner beliefs, so we can realign them with our emotions in a healthy, useful way."[71]

For example: when I am six months old and hungry, if nobody sticks a bottle or a breast in my mouth, it is primal instinct for me to start yelling to express my emotion. There is no thought there, just the raw emotion. But as I get older I can think about how to satisfy my hunger by doing something appropriate. I can ask Mommy for food or take a cookie from the cookie jar myself.

Thoughts are a bridge to us getting in touch with emotions, because we are no longer just instinctive-emotional people. As we grow up, we become thinking people. By observing and understanding what happens to us, why an experience was necessary, we can recognize unconscious feelings fueling our reaction to the experience.

Here is how the process works: Baby Jane, who has had more than her share of painful medical procedures, cries when she sees her doctors because crying is her primal, instinctive, emotional reaction. Doctor visits are often painful, scary experiences which involve shots, blood work, being poked and even manhandled, so crying becomes her habitual reaction.

As Jane gets older, her unconscious belief (doctors hurt me) will determine her behavior—until she recognizes it. On a conscious level she may experience a reluctance to go to doctors and not know why. But she may be justifying her emotional reaction to doctors with the unconscious seedthought, "Doctors are people that hurt me." If Jane can recognize that the doctor was there for her good, even though the shot felt painful, she can modify her actions based on her new understanding. Instead of the unconscious knee-jerk avoid-doctors reaction, Jane will respond to doctors more appropriately.

A more helpful thought for Jane would be, "True, those doctors caused me pain when they worked on me, but it was for my own good. I don't need to fear doctors anymore." Her primal emotion of fear is accepted. But the seedthought "doctors hurt me," which was a rigid core belief as an infant, is not valid in the present. Understanding this, she is freed to be helped by her doctors.

Dis-ease is related to unconscious feelings which could be expressed in words such as "I'm not good enough," "I don't love myself enough" or "I'm not worthwhile." The accompanying unconscious core belief: "I'm not good enough" is generally based on forgotten childhood decisions such as: "Teacher yelled at me. I'm feeling bad so I must be bad."

Life experiences trigger our emotional memories. Sometimes these memories are warm and pleasant and we are happy to remember them. Other memories may be negative and unpleasant. We can allow ourselves to feel them or avoid feeling them. Substance abuse, drinking, overeating, and overmedicating are among the classic ways people avoid feeling their feelings.

When a memory triggers a negative emotion your thoughts tell you, "I can justify feeling this way because of a whole slew of reasons derived from past experiences." If you don't change the original "I don't love myself" programming you justify having and misusing the present-day emotion. You'll take a trip down memory lane reminding yourself of all your past negative beliefs, trapping yourself in a quagmire of unhealthy thoughts. You'll not have a chance to deal with your emotion constructively. You'll say or do something unwise. In the extreme case some such negative thoughts can even lead to destructive impulses, which result in murder or suicide.

It is possible to transform unhealthy, negative thoughts and feelings. Looking for the lesson to be learned from a past experience is often helpful.

In order to change the meaning of the original feeling you must first be conscious of it. Start paying attention to the interior dialogue which validates your feelings. Then you must re-examine the beliefs you've built up from your past experiences with that feeling. You'll need to recognize your own goodness: "Even though teacher yelled at me and I felt awful, that doesn't mean I'm bad. I am good enough." The changed dialogue leads to new inner beliefs. You will have rid yourself of the primal emotion as a negative force in your life and turned it to your advantage.

Underlying most negative emotion is fear of one sort or another. Unrealistic fears are potentially harmful and among the easiest to release or transform. For example, some people develop excessive fears about going to the dentist. Others fear talking in public. They have not come to terms with their original emotional reactions to such events and released their fear. But they can! Once a stressful earlier event has been uncovered, people are able to bring later learning and adult insight to bear on it. The best way to pacify your emotions is to learn something from them.

Emotions exist. They are always there. Will they run you? Or will you use their energy to build yourself a happy life? The quality of your life is determined more by interior states than by external circumstances. To feel well, your emotional as well as your physical digestive system must be in tip-top working order. The seedthoughts that you plant based on your past experiences will determine whether you will be positively or negatively affected in the present. The good news is that the choice is yours!

Self-Help Experience # 14

Witnessing Practice: Paying Attention to Yourself

Purpose: To expand self-knowledge. Practicing observing yourself as if you were another person leads to greater objectivity and honesty with yourself.

Instructions:

1. *Throughout the day, observe yourself at regular intervals, while sitting, standing, or walking.* Make believe you are across the room from your body and describe what you see. Don't be discouraged if this is difficult. If you can't see yourself, pretend or imagine you can.

2. Another way to observe yourself is to feel the different parts of your body and *describe to yourself how each part feels.*

Examples:

• I am slouching as I stand.
• There is a pulling sensation in my lower back on the right side.
• I feel a cramp in my abdomen.
• My left arm is itching.
• My eyes are watering.

3. *Notice any thoughts you are having.* You might say, "I have been thinking about..." Then return to your current activity and take your attention off yourself.

4. *Consciously use your mind to tell yourself how you feel physically and emotionally at any given moment.* All of us have experience talking silently to ourselves—that incessant chatter that intrudes on our inner peace. Maybe we have thoughts like, "What if?" or "Why me?" or "How come?" or "What's wrong with him?" Just notice what you are saying to yourself. You don't have to do anything.

What isn't tried won't work.
—Claude McDonald

Self-Help Experience #15

Questions for Illness

Purpose: To investigate the source of your disease. Your typical ailments can reveal a blueprint in your system. As you observe your recurring symptoms (sore throats, pimples, stomach aches, tumors, sprained ankles), you can uncover the seedthoughts which may be triggering these ailments.

Instructions:

1. How are you feeling—right now? Describe to yourself the way different parts of your body feel, paying special attention to any uncomfortable sensations. What is your emotional state? Are you happy, sad, angry, bored, excited, curious, interested?

2. Focus your attention on your primary physical complaint. Describe it to yourself.

3. What do you believe is causing your current discomfort?

4. Ask yourself, "What is this dis-ease trying to teach me?"

5. What is going on in your life right now? Recall the past few weeks. What is ahead that you may be dreading or looking forward to?

6. Can you recall a time in the past when you felt this way or experienced similar circumstances?

7. What do you believe would help you to feel better?

It takes practice and self-discipline to understand the message of ill-health. But the reward of a happier, healthier, more contented daily life is worth the time and trouble.

To plant a garden is to believe in tomorrow.
—Breast cancer survivor

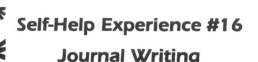

Self-Help Experience #16

Journal Writing

Purpose: To write yourself to greater awareness and self-knowledge.

Instructions:

1. Record the events of your day and note how you were feeling. Even if you generally have difficulty getting in touch with your feelings, focusing your attention on yourself by keeping a journal will encourage your true feelings to surface. Write at least once each day.

2. List who you saw, where you went, any projects you accomplished, how you generally felt during the day. It is not necessary to write complete sentences. I often use my appointment book to jot down things I want to remember.

3. Once a week, look over your notes and see if you learn anything new about yourself.

For example, to learn how different foods affect you, write what you ate and later note how you felt. Journal keeping can be used to uncover how people, places, or things affect you. When you re-read your journal over several days or weeks, you might discover that whenever you go to a certain place, or see a certain person, you get upset. Often, we know these things subconsciously, but we don't realize the truth consciously until we review our written records. The more you learn about yourself, the easier it will be to make changes.

Life does not consist mainly or even largely of facts and happenings. It consists mainly of the storm of thought that is forever flowing through one's head.
—Mark Twain

I need this like a hole in the head.

I put my foot in it.

I should keep my big mouth shut.

Read my lips.

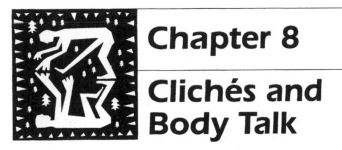

Chapter 8

Clichés and Body Talk

As children, in order to produce a magical result, many of us chanted the so-called children's gibberish words "abracadabra." I am told by more than one trustworthy source that this ancient incantation, used in many languages, is Aramaic for "I create as I speak." Little did we know then that there might be some literal truth to the idea that what we speak might come into existence.

A woman wrote Dear Abby about her beloved boyfriend, saying he does something "that simply kills me." Another common expression is "that person will be the death of me." Why do we talk like that? We mean to express emotion. But using sayings like "that kills me" to express a feeling can be dangerous. People instinctively know words hurt them when they say "I am sick—or even sick to death—of hearing about that."

Dangerous Seedthoughts

Linda Zelizer is a hypnotist and psychotherapist familiar with the power of seedthoughts. One of her male patients had a heart condition. She noted the following interesting behavior: "When he described certain upsetting incidents, he took his right hand and beat his chest, exclaiming, 'That just breaks my heart,' suggesting to his inner mind the image of a broken heart. Upon realizing this, he stopped beating on his chest and using those words. During hypnosis he gave himself positive suggestions by planting healthier seedthoughts such as 'My heart is strong and well.' His heart healed fine."[72]

Phrases like "that breaks my heart" can create an image of a "broken heart" in the subconscious part of the mind which doesn't exercise discrimination or rationality. The seedthought "broken heart" becomes an imaged pattern of beliefs embedded in the body. Frequency of use seems to increase the power of the thought to do harm. Language affects us if or when our body translates certain seedthoughts and core beliefs into physical expression.

Connecticut cardiologist, Steven Kunkes M.D. said, "Patients frequently say 'That breaks my heart' or 'I was heartbroken.' But not just heart patients!"[73] It's reassuring that many people who talk that way don't become cardiac cases. Still, there is a chance that talking that way—using provocative cliché images—can program one for bodily harm. Common sense dictates that prudent behavior would be to eliminate these potentially harmful clichés from your speech. Then *counteract any past programming* by acknowledging those things in your life that do your heart good. The way we talk may be considered another risk factor in assessing health.

Various bodily sensations like pain and muscle tension can reflect one's feeling of being burdened by life. When you feel you have too much to carry, your emotions can translate into a thought like "I can't bear it anymore."

Fairfield, Connecticut chiropractor Dr. Jacqueline Ruzga reported: "In the last six months I've had at least a dozen patients who complained, in various words, that they were 'carrying the weight of the world on their shoulders.' Every one of them had shoulder problems. Healing shoulder problems is now a specialty of mine."[74] I too felt a heavy burden as I was working on the second edition of *Your Body Believes Every Word You Say.* I developed an annoying pain in my right shoulder. It disappeared the day after I sent the first draft of the book to my editor.

Over and over I heard "Its important to listen to one's patients"[75] from other members of my medical advisory team.

Hamden, Connecticut endocrinologist Bob Lang, M.D., considers "healing conversations" an integral part of his practice. "The conversations we have with ourselves appear to affect our health. *Illness can result from ineffective conversations.* Back pain, for example, is often associated with someone saying to himself, 'I'm not being supported.' He may not recognize the implications of this thought until I point it out to him during a 'healing conversation.' *Healing is often the result of an effective conversation.*"[76]

Steven Hirshorn, M.D., a colon and rectal surgeon confirms that symptoms can disappear spontaneously after a healing conversation. He said,

"In my office, I spend more time listening to patients than doing any procedures. Frequently patients are surprised at my interest in them as people. I tell them, 'I need to know you as a whole person, not just an organ system.'

"During an initial visit with a new patient, I frequently see the symptoms disappear when the patient realizes that the symptoms are not necessarily indicative of serious illness. Occasionally a patient is in severe pain from rectal muscle spasms and while we are talking, the spasms will spontaneously cease. Later, some patients may have spasm recurrence, but just as frequently, these spasm problems do not recur. I see two things at work although the reasons for this may be more complex. I give the patient hope. And, by allaying their fears, I help them put the symptoms in their proper place, so they don't blow them out of proportion. Talking and listening are tools in my medical bag."[77]

I can confirm the value of a good healing conversation with

someone like Dr. Hirshorn. Several years ago, though I should certainly know better, I found myself frequently using the "pain in the ass" cliche to express my feelings. Eventually I began to notice distressing symptoms in that part of my body. To make matters worse, I didn't believe that anything lasting could be done to alleviate the situation. I had been led to believe that even surgery might not be successful. I definitely felt discouraged until I spoke with Dr. Hirshorn. After that initial conversation I knew that I had a viable option. Shortly thereafter the symtoms had diminished sufficiently so that no treatment seemed necessary. Once I became conscious of it, I banished the "pain in the ass" cliche through vigilant attention. The combination of altered language and viable options is potent medicine.

The Body's Messages

The body does not distinguish between our figurative and our literal language; instead it seems to mirror that which we think or speak. These next stories are true examples of people who have discovered symptoms of their bodies to be messages from their mind and emotions. See if any of these examples ring true for you. Remember that each person has his or her own unique signals.

During counseling, Paula, a former student of mine, found evidence of a seedthought that signaled her inner dissatisfaction. Her knee gave her difficulty whenever she had to face something she felt she couldn't bear. She was hanging on to an unhappy marriage and she often said, "I can't bear it." Recognizing the language connection helped Paula choose to exit the unhappy marriage and eventually create a much more satisfying one. If her knee hurts now she knows some inner self-examination is required.

Nomi's ankle was sore for two years after a minor injury. She was unable to ice skate, her favorite recreational activity. During a counseling session, she realized how often she said "I can't stand it." After she realized the connection and stopped feeding herself this negative seedthought, her ankle improved sufficiently for her to resume skating.

Another student, Bob, developed a condition similar to lock-jaw after a Novocaine injection. For three months, he could barely open his mouth. After hearing about the language connection Bob told me that he frequently had the thought, "I gotta stop talking." To those people suffering from TMJ—temporomandibular joint dysfunction of the jaw—have you ever berated yourself for talking or eating too much? Have you ever told yourself or someone else, "I wish I'd kept my big mouth shut?"

Westport, Connecticut psychotherapist and health counselor Roberta Tager provides a personal example: "Recently I was listening to some tapes of a counseling session I had with my supervisor. Self-critically I kept repeating over and over, 'I have to stop talking.' Two days later I lost my voice. Be careful what you say—you may get it!"

Tager has had other experiences of the language connection. She recounted, "Dr. Maxwell headed the admissions committee for his country club. During his term, he frequently said, 'I need this like a hole in the head.' After several years he discovered a growth on his face which left an indentation—a strange growth which looked literally like a 'hole in his head.' The indent, situated on the right side of his face between the temple and the eye, was surgically corrected. A lab report indicated that basal or cancerous cells were completely removed. He no longer uses that cliché."[78]

Sue, a former student, recounted this story: "When I was a little girl my mother and I went on a six-week overseas vacation. As we were leaving for the airport my father told me how much he'd miss me. After that leave-taking, I developed ear infections whenever I traveled by airplane, and I had no idea why. During a self-improvement seminar, I remembered responding to my father's words by thinking, 'I don't want to hear that.' The seed had been planted to 'not hear things' during plane travel. Since uncovering that seedthought and without medical treatment, I am free of the recurrent ear infections. And I travel by plane quite a bit."

Vincent Scavo, M.D., a retired ear, nose, and throat specialist, confirmed the frequency of cliché talk among his thousands of patients. He said: "You'd be amazed how many patients tell me 'I don't want to hear that!' They come to me and I'm their doctor. I shoot straight from the hip. But they don't want to hear when I tell them the truth."[79]

Chest specialist David Bushell, M.D., said: "My patients often say 'There is something I have to get off my chest.' I am not sure what if anything the connection is to their disease, but I hear the metaphor a lot."[80] *People speak their feelings both mentally and physically.* Different people have different parts of their body through which they tend to express emotions. Yet it stands to reason that individuals might focus their mental and emotional energies in the same place. So one's words and bodily symptoms tend to be related metaphorically.

Dr. Hirshorn, the colon and rectal surgeon, said, "I hear the 'pain in the ass' metaphor so often. One of the most common jokes in my office is how frequently our patients say 'I am sorry, I know I am being a pain in the ass' and then they laugh ha ha ha."[81]

Emily, a professional woman, talked of getting terrible headaches whenever she wore her new glasses. The doctors could find no organic reason for these headaches. She said, "Since I could not see well without my glasses, I went for counseling to see if I could find a psychological reason for my headaches. My therapist asked me, 'What is it you don't want to see?' I realized the truth of that question. There *was* something I didn't want to see. I faced the problem and now am able to wear my glasses comfortably. Now I want to see!" Not everyone has such rapid success.

Psychotherapist Linda Zelizer said:

"A client of mine was having violent arguments with her husband. She realized that her eyesight began to fail when she made the decision, 'I don't want to see that.' The woman labeled this a coincidence. She believed her failing eyesight was a physical problem only and refused to consider the possibility that it might have another element. When I tried to make her aware of the mental/emotional component she became angry and resistant, and stopped treatment.

"I find many people have difficulty with the connection between their body and their words and thoughts. I stress to them that these statements were made without their awareness of the possible consequences of such talk. They are then offered the choice of being responsible for themselves or remaining victims. Many, like this woman with the failing eyesight, seem more comfortable in the role of victim. They refuse to recognize a link between what they think and say, and how they feel.

"Another patient had lost his voice. During therapy he recalled that after an argument he had had the thought, 'Telling people what you think can ruin a relationship.' By losing his voice, he insured that he could not say what he thought. He was shocked when he realized he had caused himself laryngitis. He acted on this realization by learning to express himself more appropriately in a caring, yet assertive way. His voice returned in a month."[82]

Ellen was complaining about her pilonidal cyst, a congenital cyst at the base of the spine that can get infected. It can be surgically removed. She told me her cyst got worse each month during her period. I asked her, "Did you ever have the thought that 'having your period was a pain in the ass?'" She gasped as the significance of this idea clicked in for her.

A few months before we were scheduled to go to press with this book, I developed a large, fluid-filled lump (bump) on my right ring finger. It was diagnosed as a digital mucus cyst, a benign though sometimes annoying and painful condition. It drained on its own. In order to cure the cyst and prevent its recurrence, outpatient surgery was suggested.

Though the surgery was considered minor, it was unclear how many days I would miss working at my computer. Since I had so much work to *handle* including finishing this book, the uncertainty caused me much stress. That greatly increased my discomfort as the cyst once again grew larger. Finally, I made up my mind that it was not going to stop me and it didn't. I canceled the surgery. When I gave myself the extra time to handle my work, I relaxed, the bump got smaller and it stopped bothering me.

Dr. Carl Gruning, SUNY College of Optometry associate professor, provides an example of how treating the physical condition can alter the mind set.

"One of my patients, a young boy, came to me because he had difficulty concentrating while reading. His ability to focus was impaired and one eye often drifted out—'walleye' in layman's terms. He was referred to me for vision training in the hope of improving his reading ability and concentration. He expressed his problem in these terms, 'My mind drifts off when I am reading.' During his vision-training program he learned how to coordinate and focus his eyes and properly integrate the visual system with the rest of his body. His focusing improved markedly after completing the vision therapy. He reads comfortably with improved comprehension. Commenting on the results of his treatment he said, 'My mind rarely drifts off now.'"[83]

Anne, a friend who is a psychotherapist, took care of her emotionally sick daughter for six months. Later she told me she was angry at her daughter for being sick, but couldn't say anything to her. During that time, a lump developed in Anne's breast. She required a mastectomy to "get it off her chest."

Jane, speaking during a support group meeting, said she often woke up in the morning with her teeth clenched, feeling afraid of something or other. She required lots of dental work. Jane wondered if there was a connection to her oft-repeated statement, "That sets my teeth on edge."

Bruce Ritter, the now deceased founder of Covenant House, a refuge for kids in trouble, once opened a fund-raising letter with these words. "If I have to tell the six-kids-that-started-Covenant-House story one more time 'I'm going to blow my brains out.' It's true—the story—every word of it, but I've told it ten thousand times and I'm sick of it."[84] I think Ritter's word's are "mind-blowing." I wrote him pointing out the danger of such talk and suggested that he stop writing, thinking, and speaking like that. Apparently, many people had written him, upset at what he'd written. He wrote back that he had merely meant to express emotion. He didn't think then about the literal meaning of his words.

Mixed Messages

A mixed message is a statement or phrase that uses both positive and negative images. Examples are expressions like: "I am pretty upset" or "That was terribly nice." When you hear the words "terrible" and "nice" together, which word do you respond to? Mixed messages can lead to mind-body communication disruptions.

Some words themselves contain mixed messages. *New York Times* columnist William Safire calls them *"Janus or two-faced words."*[85] Janus was a Roman God with two faces. Awe, for example, is defined by Webster as "fear mingled with admiration or reverence." When someone says "I feel awful" he usually means something negative. But awe-ful in the sense of being inspiring or filled with awe could "arguably" be positive. In fact, several hundred years back, in Queen Anne's time, awful was considered a royal compliment. Now the meaning has flip-flopped and the phrase "I feel awe-ful" is an expression of discomfort. As Safire wrote, "If words exist to communicate meaning, Janus words are not good words. They communicate confusion."[86]

"I'm sorry, I feel so bad," or "I feel terrible about that" are words used when apologizing to another, or in expressing sympathy, regret, or remorse. The speaker often doesn't feel bad at all but merely wants to express herself in a forceful way to prove she is genuinely sorry. A sympathizer might say the expected "I feel so badly" and not mean it or really care what's happening to the other person.

Telling yourself or another person that you feel bad can trigger such feelings in body and mind. It's a lie, which is bound to have repercussions: *your words and feelings are in conflict.* It is unwise to affirm "I feel bad" when you mean it as an apology, because those words are often perceived by the body as an order for uncomfortable physical feelings. Such common expressions convey to your unconscious mind a set of instructions which can cause dis-ease.

Rx: Positive Talk, Positive Thoughts, Positive Attitudes

We can deliberately create helpful seedthoughts. There are phrases common to our language which can help us without our realizing it. For example, Mr. Niles, a former Tager client, was given only a few months to live after being diagnosed as having pancreatic cancer. Two years later, he was doing extremely well. According to Tager, he often says, "I don't let anything bother me anymore."[87]   His words indicate a positive attitude which reduces the effect of stressful emotions and supports the efficacy of his chemotherapy treatments. To paraphrase my teacher Dr. Ellerbroek, *It isn't what happens that makes you sick, its what you tell yourself about what happens that dis-eases you.* Don't Worry—Be Happy. Plant positive seedthoughts!

Through the enlightened use of language we can often reverse the consequences of prior abuse. Remember Abra Cadabrah—"as I speak I create." Obviously we do use language positively quite often. Notice the balance between your use of positive and negative seedthoughts. It is well worth the effort to prescribe for yourself a *feast* of positive, health-affirming thoughts and words and a *fast* from the negative, dis-easeful ones.

Self-Help Experience #17

Verbal Hygiene I

Purpose: To be aware of clichés and other expressions you may use unconsciously.

General Instructions:

Read through the following lists. Do you use any of these expressions? Ask yourself what emotion you really meant to express. Can you think of a better way to express that feeling? Notice which clichés are most familiar to you. Do they feel right? Perhaps some of them are seedthoughts for you. Ask yourself what effect these sayings might have on your body. Practice verbal hygiene—think before you speak. Cancel or erase those expressions you use which might be unhealthy. Verbal hygiene cleans up your mental act by cleaning up your thoughts and words. Think, speak, and act in ways that prevent disease from occurring physically.

Emotional Phrases, Clichés & Seedthoughts

I get choked up with emotion.
I cried my eyes out.
I'm a nervous wreck.
It blew my mind.
I need this like a hole in the head.
I need to get this out of my head.
I must get this off my chest.
I've got to stop eating.
I let my body go to pot.
I feel stuffed.
I can't stomach him.
I can't digest that.
I got cold feet.
I lost my nerve.
I froze with terror.
I wish I was dead.
I put my foot in it.
I went off my rocker
I went crazy.
I flipped out.
I nearly died.
I fight:
    for attention;
    for what I believe in;
    for my rights.
I blew:
    it;
    my cool; my stack.
I feel:
    like a square peg in a round hole;
    all tied up.
I'm a glutton for punishment.
I can't:
      bear it anymore;
      think straight;
      believe it;
      see straight.
I got ambushed (surprised) by a disease, a circumstance.

(continued) next page

I'm sorry: I feel so bad;
I feel terrible about that.
I am:
    breaking out;
    burning up;
    itching to get going;
    spaced out;
    uptight;
    sick and tired of;
    sick to death of;
    scared to death of;
    petrified—rigid, frozen, unable to act;
    frozen with fear;
    eaten up with anger;
    in a stew over that;
    heart broken;
    torn apart;
    stiff as a board;
    out of my mind with...(worry, fear, grief);
    in a dead-end situation;
    dead on my feet;
    not good enough;
    too good for you;
    at the boiling point;
    overcome with emotion.
I am dying to:
    retire;
    do that;
    get that;
    see that;
    ...and so on.
That:
    was a pain in the neck;
    gives me a headache;
    breaks my heart;
    drives me crazy;
    will give me a heart attack;
    will be the death of me;
    makes my blood boil;
    tears my guts apart;

rips me apart;
just kills me;
makes me sick to my stomach;
sets my teeth on edge;
makes my skin crawl;
is hard to swallow;
weighs on me;
is nerve wracking;
is a bitter pill to swallow.
There's a knot in my stomach.
Something is eating away at me.
My heart feels shut down.
My mind drifts off.
My feet are killing me.
It is:
eating at my gut;
a pain in the ass;
just my luck;
in my blood.
My nerves are raw.
What an unnerving experience.
The crisis reached a head.

If a picture is worth a thousand words, please
paint me the Gettysburg Address.
—Leo Rosten

Self-Help Experience #18

Verbal Hygiene II: Group Seedthoughts

Purpose: To uncover some prejudices and widely held beliefs.

Use these lists to assist you in observing your mind. Your thoughts and words are indicative of your beliefs. Then con-

(continued) next page

sciously decide: "Are these ideas really true for me? Do I want to hold on to these beliefs?" Some of these are clichés, some are seedthoughts, and some are not. But all represent a definite set of beliefs held by various groups of people.' Sometimes, in your conscious mind you may reject an idea. But if you have heard it often enough, any of the following ideas may actually be part of the fabric of your unconscious belief system. You could be affected by them without realizing it. Truly, the examined life is most worth living. Add to these lists on your own.

Which of the following statements do you have lurking in the depths of your mind, like time bombs or mines waiting to explode? Some of them like "Honesty is the best policy" might even be good for you. But let it be your conscious choice now to keep them.

Health-Related Beliefs:
Old age brings illness.
Only the good die young.
Cancer, stroke, or heart disease cause death.
AIDS is always fatal.
Disease attacks regularly through life—there is little that can be done about it. Sickness is inevitable.
That disease (cancer, stroke etc.) runs in my family.
That was the straw that broke the camel's back.
Without medicine that (disease) can't improve.
You must move your bowels once a day.
I'll die at the same age as my parents.
No pain no gain.
An apple a day keeps the doctor away.
Grin and bear it.
Blow a gasket.
Blow my brains out.
Roll over and play dead.
I should have my head examined.
I did it just for the hell of it.
I need to 'spill my guts.'
Cry yourself to death; laugh yourself to health.

Stress:
> can kill you;
> is bad for you;
> is good for you.

I was caught off guard.
Ignorance is/is not bliss.
What you don't know won't hurt you.

Prosperity, Work, and Sex-Related Beliefs:
Money is power.
You need to have money to make money.
More of "anything" is better. Less is more.
Men are more interested in sex than women.
All men care about is sex.
Women take forever to come.
Women use sex to "control" men.
Men use money to "control" women.
What you resist persists.
Seeing is believing.
What you sow you reap.
What goes around, comes around.
Honesty is the best policy.
When the going gets tough, the tough get going.
Better late than never.
You just can't win.
It's a no-win situation.
A stitch in time saves nine.
I'll be the first one laid off, you wait and see.
It always happens to me.

Eating Metaphors—Food for Thought:
Now you're cooking.
Feed your mind.
Hungry for sex.
Eat your words.
Chew on it.
Swallow your pride.
You're full of it.
That has a bite to it.

(continued) next page

Eating:
    too much is bad;
    too little is bad.

Superstitious Beliefs—Common Sayings:
Good things always come with bad.
Things, good or bad, happen in threes.
Friday the 13th is a bad luck day.
Don't walk under a ladder.
Step on a crack, break my back.
Don't let a black cat cross your path.
Garlic around the neck wards off evil.
Cross your heart and hope to die.
Cross your fingers—to allow you to lie.
Cross your fingers—for good luck.
See a penny pick it up, all day long you'll have good luck.
Let sleeping dogs lie.

Relationship-Related Beliefs:
Being competitive brings out the beast in us. Being coopera-
    tive brings out the best in us.
Revenge is sweet.
Change is easier if not changing carries a price.
Women/girls are better at....
Men/boys are better at....
Girls drive me crazy.
Boys drive me crazy.
Good guys finish last.
If you don't have something nice to say, don't say it.
Why is everybody always picking on me?
Never trust:
    a woman;
    a man.
Never trust anyone:
    over thirty;
    under thirty.
There is something inherently wrong or sinful with everyone
(to some the bible posits this concept of original sin).

If the facts don't fit the theory, change the facts.
—Albert Einstein

Self-Help Experience #19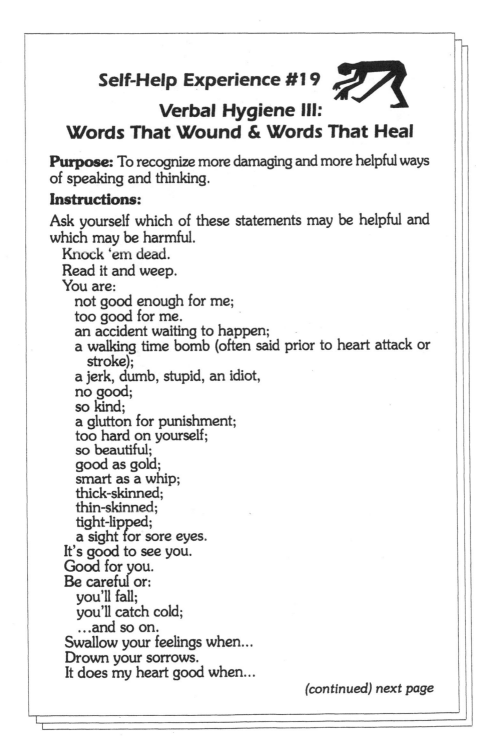

Verbal Hygiene III:
Words That Wound & Words That Heal

Purpose: To recognize more damaging and more helpful ways of speaking and thinking.

Instructions:

Ask yourself which of these statements may be helpful and which may be harmful.

Knock 'em dead.

Read it and weep.

You are:

    not good enough for me;

    too good for me.

    an accident waiting to happen;

    a walking time bomb (often said prior to heart attack or stroke);

    a jerk, dumb, stupid, an idiot,

    no good;

    so kind;

    a glutton for punishment;

    too hard on yourself;

    so beautiful;

    good as gold;

    smart as a whip;

    thick-skinned;

    thin-skinned;

    tight-lipped;

    a sight for sore eyes.

It's good to see you.

Good for you.

Be careful or:

    you'll fall;

    you'll catch cold;

    ...and so on.

Swallow your feelings when...

Drown your sorrows.

It does my heart good when...

(continued) next page

Smile and the world smiles with you.
Share and share alike.
It never hurts to be nice.
Read my lips.
Eat your heart out.
Bite your tongue.
It's just not fair.
You will never amount to anything.
Why did I say that?
Swallow your pride.
I couldn't do that.
I'm afraid not.
I hate you.
I love you.
If only...
What if...?
Why me...?
Keep on keeping on.
If at first you don't succeed, try, try again.
When the going gets tough, the tough get going.
You're not yourself today. You don't look good.
You look:
   tired;
   sick;
   wonderful;
   handsome;
   beautiful.
It ain't over 'till the fat lady sings.
Make the best of it.
Make the most of it.
Expect the best. Prepare for the worst.
This too shall pass.
Move traffic in the direction it's going.
Out of the mouths of babes often comes wisdom.
An ounce of prevention is worth a pound of cure.
Count your blessings.
Every day in every way I'm getting better and better.
I wish you many blessings.
Heaven Help Us.

*Every tomorrow has two handles. We can take hold of it with
the handle of anxiety or the handle of faith.*
—Henry Ward Beecher

Self-Help Experience #20

Releasing Painful Emotion

Purpose: To get over hurt feelings and prevent the need to get a physical illness to express your emotion.

Instructions:

1. *Acknowledge* your hurt, but don't dwell on it. The longer you dwell on an emotion, the more at home you feel, and the more likely you are to induce illness.

2. *Express* your hurt feelings in positive ways, like crying, talking or writing it out.

3. *Find* ways to nurture yourself with positive activities like exercising, taking a bath, having a massage, doing something creative, artistic, musical or even eating a piece of chocolate!

4. *Remove* negative thoughts by replacing them with more positive ones. Think something as simple as, "It does my heart good to see a rainbow, or listen to music, or eat a good meal (or whatever you like to do)." Even if you are deeply unhappy you can find something that makes you feel good.

5. If you find yourself dwelling in self-pity, whether justified or not, remembering other people in worse circumstances is sometimes helpful.

If you want to get to the kernel, you have to break the shell.
—Recovered mental health patient

You see what you believe.

It never rains but it pours.

I should live so long.

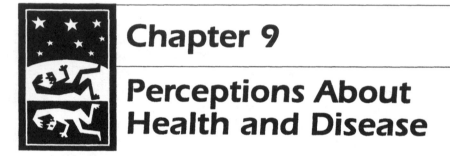

Chapter 9

Perceptions About Health and Disease

Our beliefs about the way things are shape the way we see things. Award winning Connecticut educator Bob Gillette has said, "When you hear a siren it can mean something terrible happened, but to the person in need of emergency assistance the siren is a wonderful sound which says 'help is on the way.'"[88]

Do our beliefs influence the way events turn out? The notion that prophecy can be self-fulfilling has some scientific truth. Researchers in perception have demonstrated that *we often see what we expect to see, hear what we expect to hear, and feel what we expect to feel.* Daily, news stories provide examples of this. We may all hear the same words or read the same story, but how we interpret it, what it means to us, comes from our underlying beliefs.

Your race, nationality, cultural, political and religious beliefs even your age predispose how you will view a given event. The twentieth century has had its share of defining events that divide people according to their core beliefs. Consider Oliver

124

North of Iran-Contra fame: Was he traitor or patriot? Your answer to this question depends on what you believe about a whole variety of issues. Most conservatives view North as a hero and most liberals see him as a traitor. Or Yasser Arafat: is he terrorist, freedom fighter, or statesman? Perhaps to some he is all three.

Over time these names may be forgotten to be replaced by others who represent different points on the broad spectrum of political or social values expressed by our core beliefs.

Consider O. J. Simpson: Did he get away with murder, or was he the victim of a "rush to judgment," evidence tampering, or police misconduct? Here too, your answer seems to depend on what you believe about a host of issues. And sad to say, the color of your skin often appears to influence what you believe vis-a-vis this case. The televised scenes of reactions when each verdict was announced were markedly different among groups of black and white Americans.

During the criminal and civil trials it became clear that the life experiences of blacks and whites altered the way they felt about not just O. J. Simpson, but about the police and the criminal justice system itself. It became clear that often blacks and whites have different core beliefs, expectations and understandings about others' actions.

Throughout history defining events have divided people according to their core beliefs slowly shaping us as a people. As the twentieth century drew to a close, the events leading up to the impeachment of President Clinton again polarized America, bringing into even sharper focus ways in which beliefs shape the way we see things.

During the Clinton impeachment process the political establishment divided sharply along partisan, cultural lines. The convict/acquit fault lines tended to reverse positions held vis-a-vis President Nixon during Watergate. Core beliefs determined how each President's actions were perceived.

During the Clinton impeachment hearings, the U.S. led a bombing run on a terrorist stronghold in Afghanistan. Many of

Clinton's Congressional opponents, already primed by their core belief that Clinton was a liar, seemed sure that Clinton was using the military attack to obstruct justice and distract the country from the trial. Only the full, vocal support of the military and Secretary of Defense could persuade Clinton's Congressional opponents to even entertain the notion that the timing of the Afghanistan attack was unrelated to the impeachment process.

The general public—also sharply divided as evidenced in opinion polls—was nevertheless consistent throughout the year in its overwhelming support for keeping President Clinton in office. Pundits fiercely debated the meaning of that support.

Commentators' explanations were colored by their own underlying beliefs. Presidential opponents belittled the people for putting up with a lying president in spite of the good economy, while supporters spoke of the wisdom of the people for recognizing that there were deeper issues like invasion of privacy and prosecutorial abuse. Many people had difficulty understanding any point of view in opposition to their own. Core beliefs can be so firmly entrenched that the believer can't even see that there might be another way to view things.

We may all have witnessed the same events, even heard the same words or read the same stories, but how we interpreted them and what they meant to us, still came from our underlying core beliefs. Perceptions about the effect of President Clinton's behavior on how he was running the country and what should be done about it depended on people's core beliefs and underlying values.

Whenever what we believe comes to pass, that reinforces our core belief. *Often what we believe will be true to us, precisely because we believe it!* In order to experience a shift in attitude, we must be open-minded enough to view new evidence and change our inner beliefs. To the extent that we are aware of our beliefs and willing to suspend them, we can learn to view any event objectively.

Scientists are supposed to be searching for totally objective truths. Yet they are now beginning to realize that they design instruments and experiments in order to find certain expected effects. In other words, what they expect to find *conditions* the way they search for it. They then often find what they are looking for, since all their efforts have been directed to this end. The way we *believe* the world is, is the way we *create* it.

We actually perceive things selectively, not noticing all that enters our field of attention. To a couch potato, a switched-on TV muffles the outside world. A child, engrossed in play, won't hear his mother call him for dinner. A cat stalking a mouse does not hear sounds it could not miss before the mouse appeared. Indeed, as Daniel Goleman, Ph.D., says in *Vital Lies, Simple Truths*, "perhaps the most crucial act of perception is in making the decision as to what will and will not enter awareness. This filtering is carried out before anything reaches awareness; the decision itself is made outside awareness."[89]

You don't just see with your eyes and hear with your ears. You also see and hear with your mind and brain. The lack of attention to new ideas and information often prevents people from recognizing and ultimately changing unhealthy beliefs.

Beliefs and the Immune System

When I am afraid because I believe I may have an illness, my thoughts put my body into a state of agitation and unrest, conditions that support the appearance of disease. But, if I believe I am healthy, I will find evidence to support that belief. I will feel more relaxed, becoming the healthy person that I believe in. Disease is allowed by the mind, even if not necessarily caused by it. Bodily conditions and seedthoughts both reflect our beliefs. In a sense, the body is a "solidified" version of the mind! Edgar Cayce, the great twentieth-century mystic and healer, summed it up by saying, "Thoughts are things and mind is the builder."[90]

How we perceive our world appears to affect our immunity to disease. Dr. Paul Pearsall relates that "Dr. Steven Locke at Harvard University Medical School found that natural killer-cell activity is diminished, not by severe changes or stressors in the life of healthy human volunteers, but by people's interpretations of stress: whether or not they see themselves as able to deal effectively with the stress that they are experiencing. It was as if immune cells behaved as confidently as the thinker in which the cells circulate. Dr. Steven Maier and associates, a University of Colorado research team, wondered whether aspects of the immune system would be responsive to "perception"—the way the brain deals with our world. They found, in their studies with rats and killer cell effectiveness, that *not being in control* results in less effectiveness."[91]

Pearsall also describes the work of Dr. Sandra Levy, who found that women treated for breast cancer show more effective killer cell activity if they are agitated than if they are resigned to their fate. Clearly, how we think and feel about what happens to us has a direct effect on our health. Believe in the strength of your body and it will reward you.

"It is not just stress or life pressures that affect our immunoefficiency, but our perceptions of our world as well... Researchers now know that cells within the immune system and within the brain itself have receptors on them that allow for interaction between the immune system and the brain. Every thought and every feeling we have alters the immune system, and every challenge to the immune system alters the way we think and feel."[92]

Flexible Thinking Creates Flexible Bodies

Many years ago, psychotherapist Roberta Tager was diagnosed as having multiple sclerosis, or MS, a degenerative disease of the central nervous system in which hardening of tissue occurs. She describes her experience this way:

"I saw some of the subconscious patterns that had shaped me, causing my disease. My thinking was rigid; my focus on the proper way to do most things was narrow. I wasn't aware that there were options in any situation.

"When I was first sick, something as mundane as being locked out of my house threw me off balance. If an obstacle arose I was almost *paralyzed, I was frozen in place.* My emotional energy would build up as I needed to find a solution. When none presented itself I felt my energy turn in on me. I felt frazzled! The energy going down my spine burned. There was no place for this energy to go, no way for me to use it. I believe that had a literal effect on my nervous system: frazzling and frying the nerves, and triggering my MS symptoms. Damaged nerves are less effective at transmitting movement messages to the muscles. I now understand that excess energy needs to be released in harmless ways, not turned in upon the host vehicle. The body is not designed to store excess energy, stress or emotion without eventually leading to breakdown and disease.

"Frozen thought patterns prevented my energy from being used in more creative ways. I believed life was filled with dead ends. Rigid in my thinking and often feeling paralyzed, I could not have verbalized these feelings at that time. But now I see the language connections that fueled these patterns and created my diseased body. MS is a disease with rigidity in the musculature and sometimes paralysis. For some people MS does become a dead end.

"My initial reaction to the diagnosis of MS was total fear. Fear of being crippled, paralyzed or dying an early death is a potent force. However I chose another path. I reconnected with my inner voice. It led me to release my fear of MS—and a reduction of the symptoms ensued. To all intents and purposes I have been healed, being free of signs of the disease for more than thirty years. Visualization, relaxation, vitamin therapy and mind control were part of the healing process along with my inner work: changing beliefs and opening myself to my own creativity."[93]

A lot of mental energy fed Roberta's seedthoughts and she manifested a serious physical disorder. For some people, underlying rigidity of beliefs might result in an unyielding and rigid body with other disease labels. In her case the rigid attitudes began to manifest in a process called multiple sclerosis, which could have led eventually to a total inability to act. She woke up in time.

It would be wrong to conclude from Roberta's case that all cases of MS arise from rigid attitudes. That is just one possible language connection. Nor will all people with rigid attitudes develop a major disease. Some people might just have a less flexible body. The desirable state is an ability to be open and flexible in mind and body, when such flexibility is necessary, and firm when that is required.

Your personality and your thought processes can increase or decrease your potential for contracting a disease related to the immune system. George F. Solomon, M.D., Professor of

Psychiatry at UCLA, studied female patients with rheumatoid arthritis—a disease that results from aberrant immune function. They "show more masochism, self-sacrifice, denial of hostility, compliance-subservience, depression and sensitivity to anger than their healthy sisters, and are described as always having been nervous, tense, worried, highly strung, moody individuals."[94] He notes that physically healthy relatives with rheumatoid factor—which may predispose them to developing the disease—appear to be psychologically healthier as well. It seems that a "combination of physical predisposition and a breakdown of psychological defenses leads to manifest disease."[95] One of the origins of the idea of a self-fulfilling prophecy might thus be the reality that our bodies fulfill the prophecies our minds make up.

Hypnosis and Beliefs

Hypnotherapist Linda Zelizer says:

"Sometimes people come for hypnosis to change a specific habit and a deeper issue surfaces. Although they want to change the habit at one level, they first must be willing to deal with their beliefs at a deeper level. They may have some emotional investment in not solving the problem. I have encountered many cases in which hypnosis uncovered deeper issues that had to be dealt with in order to release the unwanted condition. Amongst them are these:

• John K. wanted to stop smoking because of an advanced case of emphysema. However, at a primitive level he believed that if he stopped smoking he would be acquiescing to the demands of his wife and mother, both of whom constantly kept after him to quit smoking. Continuing to smoke had become a symbol of rebellion and freedom on a subconscious level.

• Ann C. had a heart condition and was afraid of dying. She was very overweight, and worried about illnesses associated with this condition. She often thought while she ate: 'What's the use? I don't care if I die!' In a sense she was slowly killing herself. She acknowledged that below the level of her surface symptoms, a part of her was depressed and wanted to die.

• Georgina R. was a young woman who wanted to lose weight but was terrified of being thin. She equated being thin with being sexually attractive. She had been molested by an uncle as a young girl. He frequently told her he couldn't resist her because she had such a lovely body.

These cases illustrate how core beliefs affect surface issues and might prevent them from being dealt with. When you get in touch with the underlying beliefs, you cope better with the feelings they engender. You can consciously decide for yourself whether any deeply held belief is still true or useful to you.

John might harmonize his fear of being controlled with his desire to live and decide to stop smoking in spite of the power struggle with the women in his life. He might tell himself, 'They aren't trying to control me, they are sharing their love for me. They just want me to live.' Ann should explore the roots of her depression and then decide if death is what she wants. Coming to grips with the depression will free her to deal with her weight and illness anxieties. Georgina must recognize and accept her feelings related to being molested and then ask herself: 'Do I want that awful incident to rule my life? Do I have to be fat to protect myself from men.'"[96]

Pre Menstrual Syndrome

There are many other examples of self-fulfilling prophecies. Consider the explanation that some women offer for irritability at a certain time each month. Right before menstruation many women ride an emotional rollercoaster, experiencing the dreaded reactions and tension of PMS. PMS symptoms evoke phrases such as "I expect my period any minute now." During menstruation women often say "Well, I have my period," words meant to excuse any untoward disturbing, irritating, or obstinate behavior. This language reflects a widely held belief that when women are in the menstrual part of their monthly cycle, they don't act rationally and they should be excused for their behavior then.

The physical changes that occur monthly are real and PMS may well be accompanied by horrendous behavior. Nevertheless how much do our words affect the experience? Are they cause or effect? *Which comes first: the experience or the belief?* When women accept as inevitable the condition called PMS, they doom themselves to experiencing it. A better approach is to look for thoughts contributing to or triggering it, in addition to using the many medical techniques now available to help manage this condition. Since this condition was first recognized many effective natural treatments have also emerged to help women suffering from severe PMS. It's important to add here that not all women suffer from PMS.

If we see menstruation as a time when our negative programming is closer to the surface, we can use this time of the month as an opportunity to recognize and then alter such programming. Menstruation brings things that are normally buried out into the open, where they can be seen on a conscious level, and so healed.

I'm Gonna Live Till I Die!

My friend Debby told me about her Uncle Harry. He frequently said "I'm never going to live to be fifty," indicative of his lifelong belief that he would die before his fiftieth birthday. During routine gall bladder surgery the day before his fiftieth birthday, Uncle Harry died on the operating table. Another friend, Judy, often spoke of her antipathy to aging saying, "I don't want to grow old." She died in a car accident shortly after turning fifty. While talking about the possibility of his son beating him at tennis Mike often said: "Over my dead body." Sad to say he died shortly after his son beat him on the tennis court.

It has been widely reported that Elvis Presley believed that older performers like Bing Crosby and Rudy Vallee had degenerated into caricatures of themselves in their primes, doing the same things they'd done years before. His seedthought was, *"I'll never let that happen to me."* He died at age forty-two, never having had the chance to age more gracefully.

When you expect to feel good, your positive attitude helps create it, no matter what the circumstances. Not always, but usually, expecting the best paves the way for the best to occur. To expect the worst paves the way for the worst to be realized. The notion behind a self-fulfilling prophecy is the concept that *what we believe is what comes to pass.* Self-awareness and honest self-evaluation of your core beliefs—after bringing them to the surface—are keys to a healthy life and a well-functioning body.

Self-Help Experience #21
I Believe...

Purpose: To uncover your beliefs.

Make a list. Start with the statement,"I believe..." You fill in the blanks. Work on your list a few minutes a day. You will soon have a rather long list. Keep a pencil beside your bed. I often awake at night with another belief to include on my list.

Sample Belief Statements:

Which, if any, of these statements are true about you?

- I am lovable and kind.
- My body feels good enough.
- I think healthy thoughts.
- I think for myself.
- I am committed to getting well.
- People often help me.
- A higher power looks after me.

- I am selfish and self-centered.
- I often feel bad.
- I often think negatively.
- I let the doctor decide.
- I'll never get well.
- People are out to get me.
- I'm alone in a hostile world.

Using the above model, create your own set of statements to uncover your beliefs about any area of your life that you want to understand better.

Some Typical Group Stereotypes:

Every group, race, religion, or nationality is subject to prejudices. Prejudices adhere whether one is male or female, young or old, black, brown, yellow or white, hetero or homo sexual and descended from one or many ethnic groups.

Following is a small sample of common beliefs used against specific groups of people. Since I dislike spreading these prejudicial words, I have deliberately left a blank space next to each. You fill in the blanks......to uncover your biases or prejudgments.

Instructions:

Pay attention to your reactions as you read through the list.

(continued) next page

Notice if you believe a specific group fits the bill and fills in the blank. Are such stereotypical ideas helpful or harmful, fair or unfair?

......are money hungry.   ......dress funny.
......are frugal.   ......wear strange hair styles.
......are stingy   ......have all the luck.
......are national fanatics. ......lie and cheat.
......are religious fanatics. ..... are good dancers.
......are poor students.   ......are great athletes.
......are dumb.   ......are hard working.
......are lazy.   ......are smart.
......are tough.   ......are untrustworthy.
......are loud and brash.   ......are inscrutable.
......are cold.   ......are great looking.
......are crooks.   ......control the media.
......are over-sexed.   ......control international finance.
......are under-sexed.   ......want to control the world.
......are good lovers.   Never trust......
......drink too much.   You can't trust....
......don't drink much.   You can always trust.....

They......(any group but your own)......aren't as good, smart, nice etc. as we (your group............) are.

Falsehood is invariably the child of fear in one form or another.
—Aleister Crowley

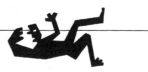

Self-Help Experience #22

Making Believe Via Creative Imagination

Purpose: To practice changing your current circumstances by directing your mind; using thought power to generate better physical and emotional health.

I've imagined getting things all my life. Often, like most of us, I have imagined the worst outcome. Now, I use imagination with greater awareness of my mental power. When I realize that I am picturing the worst, I cancel the negative scenario and replace it with a more desirable one. This process works well for me.

For example, two years after my brain surgery, I was given a surgical option for improving my voice by injecting a surgical Teflon into my paralyzed vocal cord. This would expand and stiffen the paralyzed left cord, allowing the right working cord to reach and vibrate against it, improving the quality of my voice. But I was still hoping the nerve would regenerate causing the cord to move. Teflon would preclude that option. While searching for the right doctor to help me, I frequently wished there were some other way to move the cords closer together. I often thought, "Why can't they just put something near my paralyzed cord in order to move it over so the good one can reach it."

Imagine my astonishment when I was told about a new operation, developed in Japan, that uses a small piece of plastic to press the paralyzed cord permanently closer to the working one. The operation was performed and my voice improved considerably.

You can make believe to encourage your chances of achieving any desired result. While completing the first edition of this manuscript and waiting for acceptance by a publisher, I often imagined myself receiving a phone call from the publisher telling me, "I loved your book and want to publish it." I made up details of the conversation and even placed a bottle of champagne in my refrigerator to celebrate when I received the call. Since you are reading this book, you know I was successful.

Instructions:

Think of a situation in your life that is consistently negative; one you want to change. Visualize the outcome you want. For example: If you want to lose weight, see yourself thin. Pretend you are eating less of the fattening foods. Compliment your-

(continued) next page

self for choosing to eat wisely. Make believe you are exercising more. Make up or imagine a scenario that will encourage modification of your former fat-inducing behavior. If you begin to eat less food and exercise more, you will certainly lose weight.

When you make believe, you are pretending something is so. Often that will motivate you to enact new behaviors and attitudes that are necessary to success. Making believe is a way to make real your consciously chosen healthy beliefs. The positive thoughts and feelings generated will have a positive physiological effect on you. You will be encouraged to think and act differently.

You can also imagine a desired outcome over which you don't appear to have any control. Often, you will generate the desired result anyway, like my vocal cord enhancement surgery. A classic example happens when you drive to a place where parking is usually difficult. Somehow, if I expect to get a parking space, I do. Some people call this sort of thing coincidence. But, expectation does seem to shape reality.

> *Imagination is the highest kite one can fly.*
> —*Lauren Bacall*

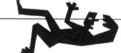

Self-Help Experience #23

Take a Stand

Purpose: To practice speaking in a creative, self-generating way to achieve results. You take a stand by saying something is so and committing to it through your words and thoughts. You aren't lying, you are creating anew, using your will and imagination to pretend and make believe until you alter your reality. You are living in faith rather than in circumstances.

Instructions:

1. *Choose* a situation that you desire to change, even a seemingly hopeless one. Declare your stand.

2. *Notice* any block to achieving your result. Do what you can to remove it. There may be nothing you can do.

3. *Express* confidence in the final outcome, often and aloud. Ask someone to agree that you will achieve your desired result.

4. *Remove* your attention from current circumstances. Focus instead on the desired end result.

5. *Recognize* that there is a higher power at work in your life. So, give thanks for any signs of progress.

6. If it doesn't work out as you desired, recognize and accept that *some things just aren't meant to be.* Ask yourself, what have I learned from the experience?

> *Confidence is contagious. So is lack of confidence.*
> *—Vince Lombardi*

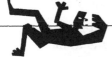

Self-Help Experience #24

Recognizing and Re-Thinking Unhelpful Thoughts

Purpose: To practice releasing worries by recognizing and changing seedthoughts. This exercise is useful for any upset including health concerns, money and business worries or even fear of failure.

Instructions:

1. *Separate the situation from the emotion.* What emotion are you feeling related to the upsetting situation? Is it anger, fear, frustration, envy, or something else?

2. *Notice your thoughts*: What are you telling yourself related to the upset?

(continued) next page

3. *Talk about your thoughts* with someone who can be trusted to help you transform any negative belief into a more helpful seedthought. Don't tell anyone who is going to agree with your negative self-judgment.

4. *Create a new, more positive seedthought.* For example, if you are worried about money say, "Money does not slip through my fingers, since I am so cautious. So even though my worries cost me emotionally, they have helped keep my business solvent. I admire myself for this." This sort of statement will help you see your fears in a positive, more useful context. Re-contextualizing your fears, imagining them from a new perspective, is putting a positive spin on the situation.

5. Following are *sample seedthoughts* that you can adapt to your situation.

I am confident and make decisions quickly and easily.
I handle my financial responsibilities with pleasure.
I'm a strong decisive leader and manager.
I have as much money as I need to pay all my bills on time.

*Always bear in mind that your own resolution to success is
more important than any other one thing.*
—Abraham Lincoln

Self-Help Experience #25

Positive Expectations in Negative Situations

Purpose: How many times have you said, "I am getting a cold" or "I am going to be sick"? Were you right? This exercise is designed to help you stop an illness in its tracks; to alter your unhealthy expectations.

Picture another possibility. Could you allow yourself to be wrong and not fulfill your belief? Wouldn't it be wonderful to stay healthy because you stop affirming your belief in a future illness? You can take precautions if you recognize signs that might mean an impending cold. These could include resting more, taking extra Vitamin C and zinc, avoiding dairy products for a time, eating chicken soup, gargling, taking a hot bath. Do whatever you *believe* might help you avoid a cold, but don't assume that the cold is inevitable.

Instructions:

1. Use this the next time you think you are getting some particular ailment such as a cold, sore throat, headache, upset stomach, or backache.

2. First, ask yourself if you need time off from your usual activities. Then give yourself permission to take that time, so you won't need an illness to get a day off. Take a wellness break instead. Do you need solitude or company? Take steps to fill that need without getting ill.

3. Describe to yourself how the ailment you're thinking about would make you feel. Be specific. Do whatever you need to do for your body and for your emotions to avoid this ailment.

4. Find a more favorable way of speaking about how you feel. Instead of "I am getting a cold," tell yourself, "My body is signalling me. I need some free time. I will listen to my body and take a wellness break." Take a stand for good health and you can often generate it.

5. In the event that you do get sick, take care of your body using any physical remedies you know to be helpful. Mend your mind and emotions by imagining and expecting a quick, favorable outcome, a return to health.

Reversing an unwanted situation or ailment is often a slow, difficult thing to do. Sometimes it may be necessary for the process to persist in order for you to learn something from the experience. There is no need for guilt or believing you haven't done it right. Be easy on yourself if an exercise doesn't seem to work for you. If it doesn't work for you, it may even turn out to be for the best.

> *What isn't tried won't work.*
> —Claude McDonald

See no evil, hear no evil, speak no evil.

You don't look so good.

What you don't know won't hurt you.

You're driving me crazy.

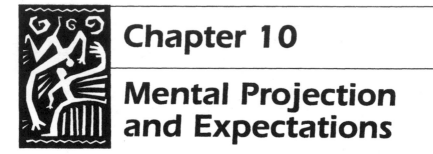

Chapter 10

Mental Projection and Expectations

By now it should be clear that your words and thoughts can affect you. But your words and thoughts also influence others, just as theirs influence you. You know the power of a smile or a few kind words to brighten someone else's day. The loving words of a friend can help you feel less stressed. Compare that feeling to the effect angry words have on you.

The words and thoughts of others affect you more than you realize. Their destructive potential is even more serious in this nuclear age. We each must be aware of what we are thinking so that our resulting words and actions will add health, love, harmony, and peace to planet Earth.

Doctors' words influence us because we tend to endow physicians with powers of knowing and healing. This is fine when they give reassurance or necessary medical advice. But there are times when doctors' words can needlessly alarm patients with negative messages. Suggestion is a powerful force through which ideas are planted in your head. Even bad news ought to be given in a positive hope-filled light.

During a workshop led by Dr. Bernie Siegel, he talked about the role of the physician in chemotherapy. Traditionally, cancer specialists warn patients to expect the unpleasant side effects of chemotherapy, including nausea and vomiting. Some prepare the patient to cope by giving instructions like, "Keep a pail beside your bed." This may be helpful advice, but it tends to generate a hypnotic expectation on the part of the patient. Often these patients fulfill the doctors' expectations by suffering side effects.

But nausea and vomiting are not the inevitable effects of chemotherapy. Quite the contrary. Many of Dr. Siegel's patients did not experience any ill effects. Since he recognized that the subconscious mind is a strong force in healing, he did not prepare his patients for suffering after their treatment. Rather, he helped them to see their treatment as a therapy which they had chosen. Those patients who recognized this choice often had less difficulty.

One patient Siegel spoke about during his workshop refused chemotherapy and radiation treatment because she viewed them as poisons—as intrusive techniques with dangerous side effects. With that attitude, she probably would have problems using the techniques, no matter how valuable they might have been. Gradually, however, she altered her thinking until she recognized radiation and chemotherapy as positive forms of energy which could help her to heal. Changing her beliefs allowed her to accept these treatments into her body with peace of mind. When she finally chose to use radiation and chemotherapy, her experience was very positive. While her body repaired itself, she felt fine, even continuing to work during the course of treatment.

Self-Fulfilling Prophecies

In describing a treatment, your doctor probably disclosed its potential side effects. I favor this as a usual procedure, especially when substantial risks are involved. These symptoms would otherwise catch you unawares and generate uncertainty and fear. But there is a real possibility that you will take your doctor's words too seriously and bring on the very side effect that you would want to avoid. You can prevent this by being aware of the effect of negative expectations and by using positive thinking.

Siegel recounts: "If I give you an injection of saline solution and say, 'Here's chemotherapy, Phil; your hair is going to fall out.' thirty percent of men will have their hair fall out."[97] One-third of women, too, receiving placebos instead of chemotherapy, will lose their hair.

Patients sometimes suffer from side effects without ever having been warned. So when a drug seems appropriate, the doctor faces a dilemma: "How do I keep the patient informed while still speaking positively?" One solution is to inform the patient within a framework of hope. The doctor might say, for example, "Some people have experienced nausea after chemotherapy, but more and more people are avoiding this unpleasant aftereffect. I believe you will be one of them."

Patients, too, are responsible and should only accept treatments they feel good about and have faith in. We have to trust both ourselves and our doctors for a treatment to succeed. Many patients are able to heal themselves and prevent or minimize the side effects of their treatment by using visualization (positive imagining) or affirmations (positive phrases) to create a mental picture of the most desired outcome.

Healing Conversations

Reducing panic—an important first step in a patient's recovery—is another way that the words of others can affect us. *Panic arises from belief in a feared outcome. Hope is belief in a desired outcome.* In a well-known story recounted in The Healing Heart, Norman Cousins spoke reassuringly to a man felled by a probable heart attack on a golf course. The man's panic subsided as he accepted Cousins's hope-filled words. Suggestion is a powerful force. Within a minute his heartbeat was slower and more regular; his color returned; he looked around and showed interest in his treatment.[98]

Dr. Jacqueline Ruzga was an emergency room staff nurse before completing her chiropractic studies. She reports:

"When a patient came in with an emergency condition—such as cardiac arrest or acute diabetic shock—a primary nursing goal was to get the patient to feel secure, comfortable, and free of panic. This agitated fear causes hyperventilation which leads to higher than normal heart rate and depletion of oxygen in the body. On more than one occasion I saw evidence of the positive effect of a loving touch and a few well-chosen, hope-filled words. 'Everything is under control. You'll be fine.'

"One patient with arrhythmia—abnormal heart rate—was in a highly agitated state. I put my hand on his back and spoke reassuringly to him. His heart rate normalized almost immediately. A young man, a victim of a motorcycle accident, was in shock, bleeding from multiple wounds. Calming the patient is an important part of slowing down bleeding. After reassurance, this man was sufficiently relaxed to have a compound fracture set without anesthesia.

"The nurse is like a surrogate mother. By touching and talking she reassures her patients, which helps to keep them alive. One man, about to undergo diagnostic tests, said he was 'frightened to death' of all the high-tech equipment around him. After some reassuring words of explanation, he went through the studies without any further problems.

"Patients need to be talked to and touched, since they often feel isolated and alone. That's why the sponge bath is such an important part of good nursing care. This warm communication between nurse and patient helps to relieve anxieties, because it tells the patient that someone cares about them; they are not alone in their time of need."[99]

Even unconscious patients need reassurance. Dr. Bernie Siegel writes, "In the operating room I'm constantly communicating with patients about what is happening, and I've found that this can make the difference between life and death. Talking to patients who are having cardiac irregularities during surgery can reverse the irregularities or slow a rapid pulse."[100] Even unconscious patients respond to words of hope and love.

At one time surgeons believed that patients under anesthesia don't hear or remember what happened in the operating room. Author Daniel Goleman describes research at a Chicago Hospital that tested the effects of words on patients undergoing back surgery.[101] While fully anesthetized these patients were given a suggestion to help them avoid the common postoperative complication of inability to urinate, which then requires catheterization to remove their urine. Not a single patient receiving the suggestion during surgery required catheterization. Suggestion is that powerful a force! Of those in a control group who heard no suggestion during surgery, more than half did require catheterization. Whether you remember hearing them or not, other people's words can affect you.

Expectations Have Power

Scary information about a disease from the media, the medical profession, and friends can influence people to hold beliefs and fears that negatively affect the outcome of the disease. *You get more upset if you expect the dire outcome.* Psychotherapist Roberta Tager says, "All illness is a group of symptoms that happen to be present at the time of diagnosis. If you name the symptoms you give power to them and they are more likely to stay with you because now you have a documented illness in which you believe. Naming can be helpful to healing by pointing to the appropriate treatment or harmful if it fosters negative expectations and an attitude of hopelessness."[102]

Multiple Sclerosis (MS) is a diagnosis that often provokes terror. Tager considers herself fortunate that so little was known about MS when she was diagnosed in 1963, as she had less negative information to dwell on. She found her own way.

Cancer is another diagnosis that still provokes terror. To many people cancer represents suffering, even a death sentence, though treatments and survival rates for cancer have improved to the point that almost every form of cancer has some long term survivors. Far from being a death sentence, cancer often gives people a chance to make positive lifestyle changes—learning to live life more fully, productively, lovingly, and joyfully.

Illness can be a powerful motivating force. It presents an opportunity for learning and personal growth, since humans often grow through the challenge of adversity. Dr. Bernie Siegel and others often talk about the gift of an illness. Learning to give and receive love is frequently an unexpected positive side effect of some illnesses. I can confirm this from my experience during brain surgery. I felt the unconditional love of my family, friends, and others.

The skillful physician communicates truthful information about your condition while maintaining optimism; something difficult to do if the doctor believes your disease is a hopeless condition. No condition, however, is truly hopeless until you are dead.

Erik Esselstyn, formerly a college dean, now a therapist, has survived bile duct cancer for over 20 years. In discussing the power of hope he said:

"When I left the hospital following surgery, chemotherapy and radiation were ruled out, being ineffective in this type of cancer. But, the surgeon gave me hope when he told me, 'Come back and see me in five years.' I reasoned, 'The doctor expects me to live if he doesn't want to see me for five years. He has set a long-term goal—way out in the future. I'll shoot for that mark.' Hope is a potent force in the healing process, a force that this capable doctor wisely activated. I remain grateful to him. Though uncertain then about my survival, I was determined to do everything possible to aid my complete healing."[103]

The Placebo Effect

Many patients respond to expectations when given pills with no intrinsic healing power, especially if they believe the pills will help them. This placebo effect is an example of a self-fulfilling prophecy. Studies of the placebo effect demonstrate the power of belief and faith in the healing process. Since people often are unaware of their true beliefs, many heal whether they think they believe in the treatment or not.

"The placebo effect in medicine is well-documented. The word is Latin from the Catholic prayer for the dead, meaning 'I shall please.' In centuries past, doctors used placebos to placate problem patients. 'You gave them something to send them away happy,' said Anne Harrington, a medical historian at Harvard University. Experts estimate that 30 percent of all patients getting placebo treatment today improve."[104]

The classic, oft-recounted case demonstrating the power of expectation in healing involved a male, advanced cancer patient. Krebiozen, a now-discredited drug then receiving widespread acclaim, was being tested at the clinic where the man was a patient. After begging for the treatment, he was given one injection by his physician Dr. West. Shortly after receiving the drug, the patient's cancerous growths "melted like snowballs" apparently freeing him from the disease. Treatment was continued with the drug three times a week till the patient was discharged. Shortly thereafter, news spread that the drug was worthless. After hearing the news and losing hope, this patient's tumors promptly recurred.

Dr. West, recognizing the powerful effect of his patient's belief system, gave him new hope when he told him that he would give him a specially prepared, more active form of the drug. For this treatment, administered with much fanfare, Dr. West in fact used a fresh water placebo. The tumors again melted away, more dramatically than before. The water injections were continued since they worked such wonders, and the patient remained symptom-free for a time. Several months later definitive studies were published showing beyond a doubt that Krebiozen was worthless. Upon learning of this, the man's tumors reappeared, and he soon died.[105]

Ronald Glasser, M.D., in *The Body Is The Hero*, reports on a paper published in the early thirties in the *Journal of The American Medical Association* by a physician who had evaluated thirty-five different published studies on the use of drugs in the treatment of high blood pressure. The author found to his surprise that every paper he'd looked at boasted either complete or significant partial relief from the material being tested. These papers variously claimed that mistletoe, diathermy, watermelon extract, even drops of dilute hydrochloric acid three times a day brought improvement in over 85 percent of the patients.

"Since all the substances tested were so radically different chemically one from the other, the author was forced to conclude that the only thing all the studies had in common was that 'the patients wanted to improve, they wanted their doctors to be successful, they wanted the drugs to work, they wanted to get better.' He attributed the successes in the studies to the well-known but little-discussed placebo effect."[106]

Glasser also reported an instance where two supposedly severely allergic patients could not be diagnosed. The patients were frustrated and angry that nothing could be found. All skin tests had been negative. A young doctor caring for them half-jokingly remarked that if only their skin tests would become positive, a diagnosis could be made, medications given and they would be cured. The next morning both patients had positive skin tests.

Minding the Body

The mind controls the body in startling ways. People with so-called multiple personalities exhibit an interesting effect. Depending on which personality is present during the testing, they have been known to change physically in mind-boggling ways. A multiple may be allergic to some substance in one personality but not in another.

Medical researcher Caryle Hirshberg and journalist Marc Ian Barasch in their well-researched book *Remarkable Recoveries* report on a young woman with multiple personalities now classified as Dissociative Identity Disorder. They wrote she "was normally allergic to grass as evidenced by her wheezing response to allergens and by skin reaction to a standard 'scratch test.' But when she was required to mow the lawn, the girl would switch into a 'boy alter' personality who displayed no such symptoms."[107]

Hirshberg and Barasch discovered impressive evidence that shifts in physiology corresponded to shifts in personality. Different researchers report clinically significant differences depending upon which "personality" was being tested in such diverse areas as eyesight variables, thyroid hormone levels, and blood pressure. They wrote, "A 1984 study found each 'personality' had distinctly different central nervous system functioning."[108]

Hirshberg and Barasch also cited a woman who had been diagnosed some years before with diabetes. "Diabetes is a disease which is normally considered a fixed condition." Yet this woman's insulin needs changed depending on which personality was in control. Her blood sugar levels were lower when she was in the sub-personality called "Sentinel." In her Sentinel sub-personality she had to alter the dosage of her insulin injections.[109]

What are we to make of such cases? How can the same body exhibit such different physiological responses? The answer probably lies in the core beliefs held by the personality in control of the body at the time that the testing was being done. *The mind controls the body in measurable ways.*

Even a developing fetus is affected by the thoughts and words of others. As we saw in earlier chapters, each emotion experienced in the mind produces its unique neuro-chemistry. These neurotransmitters produced in the brain of the pregnant woman then cross the placental barrier into the body of the developing baby. So when the pregnant woman feels shame, anger, or elation, the child's body chemistry changes to match.

The not-yet-born child responds to sounds as well as thoughts and feelings. During a TV show called "Cradle Hypnosis," psychologist John Bradshaw discussed these effects.[110] He cited the work of two Boston University researchers—Dr. William Condon and Dr. Louis Sander—who discovered that so-called random movements of infants immediately coordinated with speech. It seems that sounds heard prenatally program neuromuscular responses.

Using high-speed sound movies and computer analysis, Condon and Sander found that each infant had "a complete and individual repertoire of body movements which synchronized with speech." Every time a specific sound was made each infant responded with an individualized muscular response; whenever that sound was heard the response was always the same for that infant. Each child studied already had its own idiosyncratic responses to language. This programming began while the child was still in the mother's womb. *It is conceivable that people's lives are affected by seedthoughts planted within them during their time in the womb.* The words used in the presence of a pregnant woman can thus have far-reaching effects.

A story recently made the rounds of the Internet which anecdotally confirms that a baby hears clearly while in the womb. A member of the Panther Springs United Methodist Church in Morristown, Tennessee encouraged her 3 year old son Michael to sing to his unborn baby sister. Daily he sang "You Are My Sunshine" to his "sister in Mommy's tummy." After the birth, the baby girl was in serious condition in the neonatal intensive care unit at St. Mary's hospital, in Knoxville.

Michael begged his parents to let him see his sister so he could sing to her. But he was not allowed in Intensive Care. As his sister's condition appeared to be worsening, Michael's mother realized that if he didn't see his sister now, he might never see her alive. So she brought him to the intensive care unit and refused to leave until her little boy was allowed to sing to his sister! He sang "You are my sunshine, my only sunshine, you make me happy when skies are gray - - -" Instantly the baby girl responded, her pulse rate became calm and steady, her breathing improved and healing intensified. The next day she was sent home from the hospital. After calling the Tennessee church to verify the veracity of this story, I passed it along to my friends via email. According to the church spokesperson, the little boy did visit the hospital to sing to his sister and she immediately began improving. The little girl is now 6 years old.

Media Messages Create Expectations

Just as doctors' suggestions and explanations can enhance or hinder the healing process, media messages may provoke self-fulfilling prophecies. Consider the plight of those folks sensitive to the pollens that cause hay fever. Starting in August and lasting for months, the media report the pollen count daily. "The Pollen Count today is 5 (or 30 or 150)!" As it rises, we hear frequent predictions of how badly we are going to suffer. Sometimes we hear warnings to stay indoors.

The higher numbers are dis-easing seedthoughts. How much good does it do to let people know these numbers? Since the amount of pollen in the air varies depending on where you are, on a low-count day you might be near a higher pollen area and therefore react strongly. In this case, if you express yourself by hay fevering, you probably will have hay fever symptoms, whether you hear the pollen count or not. Constant warnings can harm those people who are highly susceptible to any hypnotic suggestion or particularly to pollen-related predictions.

I especially remember 1983 when the media described the likelihood of a terrible year for New England hay fever sufferers. They reminded us that we'd had a wet spring and a hot, dry summer that encouraged more weeds and higher pollen levels. How many people who never had hay fever experienced symptoms that year? I met a few! The pollen count is meant to be helpful. But considering the creative power of beliefs, perhaps these warnings produce the opposite of their intended result. What can one do after hearing the pollen report—wear a mask?

Given the large numbers of messages of this nature that we receive every day, it is high time all of us learned to use positive affirmations and mental imaging techniques to counteract the negative messages that we hear and read. Paul Pearsall writes about "a woman experiencing a severe hay fever reaction to pollen for twelve years. She was helped to imagine herself free of symptoms. She became completely free of her symptoms for the first time."[111]

Another distressing message was imparted by *People* magazine in its May 1989 issue. The cover story described the long-term effects of divorce on children of all ages. The statement on the cover was "Children of Divorce: Wounded Hearts." Think of the image that headline transmits: a memorable message to the subconscious mind. Frequent advertisements for this issue appeared on TV, so I bought a copy to see how powerful the message was. I found this quote on the index page. "For years, psychologists thought that divorce was something kids got over, like chicken pox. But as those children know and a recent study has confirmed, the pain of a ruined marriage may linger in a child's life for years, causing confusion and heartache into adulthood."[112] The article itself, though it presented disturbing information, ended on a rather hopeful note, but this message was subservient to the distressing headline.

You Get What You Believe

Two oft-quoted anecdotes regarding the effects of words on patients are provided by Bernard Lown, M.D., a professor of cardiology at Harvard University.[113] One woman heard her doctor say she was a classic case of T.S., which meant Tricuspid Stenosis or heart murmur—a common, non-serious condition. She was convinced T.S. meant "terminal situation." No amount of reassurance by others could reverse that belief and her doctor was nowhere to be located. She died later that same day despite determined efforts to save her.

A critically-ill heart attack patient was amazingly helped by a belief formed upon hearing his doctor's comment to the attending staff: "This patient has a wholesome, very loud third sound—gallop" (actually a poor sign that denotes that the heart muscle is straining and usually failing). The patient recovered. He said, "When I overheard you tell your colleagues I had a wholesome gallop, I figured I still had a lot of kick to my heart and could not be dying. My spirits were for the first time lifted, and I knew I would live and recover." Occasionally "ignorance is bliss." Sometimes "what you don't know won't hurt you."

The words and thoughts of those around us can influence us positively or negatively. A workshop leader told me the following story:

"As a young boy, one of my clients had rheumatic fever. He was told repeatedly, 'Don't play—you may die.' Sometimes he played and felt faint, light-headed, or dizzy. These sensations supported the warning that he could die if he played too hard. In fact, the rheumatic condition this man had was a self-correcting type that is outgrown after adolescence. However, the now unconscious seedthought, 'Don't play or you'll die' had taken root in his mind-body system as a core belief.

"When he came to my workshop he had shut down to the joy and playfulness of life. During the workshop, he discovered the seedthought which was interfering with his aliveness and ability to participate fully in life. After the workshop he became much happier and led a more productive life. You can counteract your harmful core beliefs just by being aware."

A woman named Faith gave me more evidence of the effect the words of adults have on children when she shared her story:

"When I was a little girl, I was severely bow-legged and walked pigeon-toed. My aunt told me, 'It hurts me to see that your leg isn't straight.' She then touched my leg and showed me how to straighten it and walk straighter. I loved this aunt deeply and was disturbed that she felt hurt. I thought about what she said quite often and attempted to keep my leg straight. But then, after a few days, the thoughts passed from my conscious mind and I just played and lived life normally. Several months later, my aunt noticed, and pointed out to me, that my leg was now straight. I was so thrilled to have pleased her. She didn't have to experience hurt for me anymore."

A man named Jim describes how he overcame the programming that limited him as a child:

"When I was growing up, I had difficulty walking, still falling often at five years of age. A doctor recognized the problem as Leg Perthes, a malformation of the hip joint. In the early 1940s this was not commonly diagnosed, nor were the doctors certain of the outcome of treatment. They prescribed no walking, bed rest, keeping pressure off the joint, and a full cast from my hips to my toes. Whether I would walk again was in doubt.

"I spent a year in bed, missing school till fourth grade. After the cast was removed, the last thing the doctors told my folks was, 'Encourage your son to study hard, so he can have a desk job. He will probably have difficulty with physical activity or exertion.' But my parents, especially my mother, bless her, always believed I would be perfect. So I believed it! She told me often, 'If you want something badly enough, you can have it.' She gave me faith in positive thinking.

"Today I am a soft drink distributor. My work is mostly physical: lifting, hauling, driving a truck. I play racquetball and exercise regularly. I believe that my mind can direct my body to do anything. I never take medicine, yet I haven't missed a day of work in 16 years. If I don't feel well, I rest and tell myself I will be well. Then I am well! Every few years I have a physical checkup and the doctor says, 'You are perfect.'"

Hope As Healer

Jim and Faith offer powerful testimony of the importance of being with people who believe in you and reassure you when you are feeling ill. Fear creates stress on the body. Prophets of doom upset the apple-cart of hope. As Dr. Larry Dossey, author of *Healing Words* wrote in the foreword to *Remarkable Recoveries*: "Which is worse—false hope or excessive optimism?"[114] He asks us to create room for "ethical hope," which is different from false hope. It rests on real possibilities, not fantasy.[115] Remember that hope isn't ever false, because a relaxed, trusting attitude creates a more favorable healing environment in the body. Don't ignore the reality of symptoms, check for organic causes, and expect a favorable outcome. Hope is a potent healing mechanism!

Its been said, "the truth will set you free." The truth is that *what we hear* affects *what we believe*. And what we believe affects whether we live or die, whether we are well or ill, whether we will prosper or wither on the vine.

Self-Help Experience #26

Helpful Reminders

Purpose: To practice presenting information in a more positive, useful, less inflammatory way.

Talk positively to others, using words, thoughts and images that suggest health, not disease. For example, it's better to say, "Eating vegetables and fruits will keep you healthier" than "If you don't eat right you'll get sick." The latter may be true but there is a positive way to present the information.

The mind remembers *the last few words* of a statement most vividly. How you phrase your warning statements is important. For example, it's better to say, "Remember to bring your homework" rather than "Don't forget your homework." The mind focuses on the last few words, in this case, "forget your homework." For example:

Common	**Better**
Don't get sick.	Stay well.
Don't forget the milk.	Bring some milk home.
Cross streets carefully or you'll get hit.	Look both ways when crossing streets.
Be careful or you'll fall.	Hold on tight.
Study hard or you'll fail.	Study hard and you'll pass.
You're driving me crazy.	I get stirred up by you.
You'll be the death of me.	I worry about you.
You confuse me.	I don't understand you.

As you go through today, listen to your language for negative statements. Picture whatever image works for you: a watchdog or a gardener in your mind—sitting between your brain and your mouth—watching for and weeding out negative statements and changing them to positive ones. For example, label someone as having a mind of his own rather than stubborn.

The mind is its own place, and in itself can make
heaven of Hell, and a hell of Heaven.
—John Milton

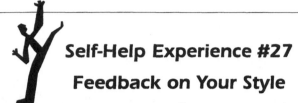

Self-Help Experience #27

Feedback on Your Style

Purpose: To recognize the effect your way of speaking has on others.

Instructions:

1. Pay attention to the effect of your words on those around you. Choose a conversation with a friend to practice on today. First, practice being reassuring in everything you say.

2. Then switch to talking negatively.

3. Notice if your listener responds differently.

4. Finally tell the other person what you were doing. Ask them for feedback on how each mode of your talking affected them.

The voyage of discovery lies not in finding new land-
scapes, but in having new eyes.
—Marcel Proust

Self-Help Experience #28

Talking With Children

Purpose: To be more aware of the ways you talk to children, so you can choose your words more appropriately.

Negative programming of young children is often glaringly apparent in waiting rooms at doctor's offices or in retail stores, especially supermarkets. I became aware of a shocking array of negative programming just listening to how parents talk to their children, especially when either parent or child is upset. For example: "Stop that or I'll kill you"; "You are driving me crazy"; "You'll never amount to anything."

(continued) next page

Instructions:

To encourage high self-esteem in children:

1. Start telling your child she *is already the way you want her to be.* For example, you might tell your baby, "You are a bright, cheerful baby." "You are handsome and friendly."

2. Pay attention to good behavior. When your child exhibits those ideals and behaviors which you value, reinforce them with praise. Don't emphasize the negative behaviors you observe. If you observe behavior you don't approve of, express your disapproval with an emphasis on the positive. Say something like, "Stop that! We prefer this...behavior instead."

3. Start now to use positive affirmations with your children, even if they are teenagers or older.

4. Believe your child can succeed in whatever he attempts. Don't berate him if he fails. Acknowledge him for trying.

5. Present your child with positive messages to enhance her self-confidence and self-esteem.

6. Encourage your child to practice making choices by offering him alternatives to choose from.

7. Expect your child to have talents and she will. The talents might not be the ones you've hoped for. Respect the uniqueness and free choice of each individual.

As you are at seven, so you are at seventy.
—Jewish Proverb

The unexamined life is not worth living.

Don't worry, be happy.

Better late than never.

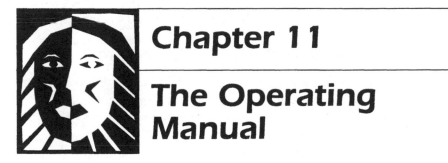

Chapter 11

The Operating Manual

Scientists in a variety of interdisciplinary fields have concluded that there is one instrument in existence with the capability of advancing civilization beyond our present-day expectations. To date, this instrument has astounded owners by its broad range of innovative uses. Because it has tremendous value to society, there is a real desire to extend its lifespan and enhance its daily operating ability. To maximize the potential of this instrument has become a primary concern of this decade.

Owners across the nation are faced with a common problem. This instrument does not come with Maintenance Instructions. Through years of ongoing experimentation, however, we have discovered that each owner must explore the available options and then create his or her own Operating Manual. Each owner is uniquely equipped to create this manual because each owner is the instrument referred to.

This instrument is, of course, the human being. We must learn how to care for this instrument if we are to maximize its potential and bring joy to its owner. Understanding mind/body communication is key. Being human is a wonderful gift!

The mind communicates with the body through language, thought, visual images, and metaphor. Seedthoughts program the body and emotions for either illness or wellness. The body talks back through physical sensations. The mind then gives these sensations meaning, providing information which stimulates more communication. This system operates continuously and automatically. A conscious mind can intervene and alter the system, for better or worse. Disease is part of the healing process.

Consciousness as Software

Human bodies are composed of billions of cells which perform a vast array of electrical, mechanical and chemical functions. The body knows very well what it is doing. It functions by being in communication with each of its parts. Body machinery continuously operates without our conscious assistance. Organs and systems such as the digestive system communicate constantly without our supervision.

Consider your body as analogous to the hardware of the personal computer. The body is the computer itself. However, something beyond the hardware (the body) is needed for the computer to operate: the software. To use my personal computer for writing I need word processing software that tells the computer what to do. As a human being you have some software built into your system, like the operating system of the computer. It's called the unconscious mind. You also have software that you generate by your thoughts, images, and words. Through your consciousness, you continuously create, revise and change programs for yourself throughout your life.

A properly programmed computer can perform functions unimaginable just fifty years ago. When programmed improperly, however, it will malfunction. Similarly, an improperly programmed human mind causes the human system to malfunction. But properly programmed and maintained, you can perform beyond what was imaginable to most people fifty years ago. Witness the new inventions created to improve the quality of life, making it easier and faster to go, to get, to do almost anything. Witness also the feats of speed, stamina, endurance, and flexibility performed during the Olympic Games.

We are only beginning to test the limits of our achievements. During the twenty-first century we may learn how to get along and trust others sufficiently to create enduring world peace. We may use our ingenuity to eradicate disease and eliminate starvation. We may travel at the speed of light. All this and more is possible for the healthy, well-maintained, finely developed human instrument. The key element in developing this potential is our level of consciousness.

Encouraging you to think for yourself, recognize your intuitive wisdom and to create appropriate software is one of the aims of this book. But thinking for yourself also means aligning your thinking towards the Higher Self, the God Self that exists for and in all of us. Thinking derived from that Self, our source of wisdom, leads to a desire for harmony and peace in the world. It leads to joining together in a common purpose for the good of all humankind.

Feedback Prevents Breakdown

Most computers have built-in feedback mechanisms which encourage internal correction before a total breakdown occurs. During a breakdown, the operator can make a correction if the malfunction is recognized in time. My first personal computer was programmed with three options I could use to prevent some data disaster—abort, retry, or ignore. These options gave me the chance to take action to avoid the disastrous loss of data.

A machine may beep or flash to alert the operator that a correction is necessary. But the human body's alert is frequently more subtle. It may be only vague discomfort, or intuition—that sixth sense—saying something is wrong. If the early warning signals are missed or misread, pain and disease often result. Disease is part of a human system's feedback. If ignored the problem may become progressively more severe.

Each part of the system gives feedback to the other parts. Your mind is the intelligence *operating* the system, and *observing* the system in operation. The system will operate more effectively and efficiently to the degree that you remain aware and observant. Your body—the hardware—will be as good as the thoughts—the software—you program in, provided you keep ridding the system of outside interference as well as internal noise, distortions, and static.

Computers are subject to distortions due to static, or "bugs" in the system. The human system is also subject to distortions (dis-ease) due to static within—stresses caused by structural problems, poor diet, toxins, putrefied waste, germs, lack of rest, harmful or unhealthy seedthoughts, and negative beliefs. Static distorts meaning in the human system, resulting in unclear communication from cell to cell, from organ to organ, and between mind and body. The human system continues to work, but static can lead to real damage in the body.

Distortion in the body affects the mind as well as vice versa. It's hard to think clearly when the body is in a weakened state. If toxins flow heavily in your blood stream, proper nourishment won't reach your brain. Poorly nourished brain cells can in turn result in unhealthy thoughts. Senility, for example, may be connected to brain cells dying from malnutrition.

Most of the chronic, degenerative diseases appear to have some of these causal relationships. The immune system, the street patrol that keeps your body cleared of invaders, needs proper physical and mental nourishment to be in tip-top shape. If the distress in your system becomes too great, you shut down for a while and must go to bed to rest while repairs are made. In more acute distress you might need hospitalization.

Both computers and humans can be afflicted by damaging viruses. To protect my PC from glitches or a major crash and consequent shutdown, I have an anti-virus program which runs automatically each day, scanning the PC system for unwanted instructions. To protect my body from illness, I strive to maintain a strong immune system by nourishing my mind, body, and spirit. My strategy involves eating healthy foods; exercising, thinking healthy thoughts; doing meaningful work to produce measureable results; going to synagogue each week, praying, talking to God, studying, meditating, listening to music, seeing movies; and making time for recreation, socializing, and fun.

Flying Blind

If I input an error into my computer, my data gets messed up. Once, while sampling a word processing program, I erased a whole disk by pressing keys whose function I didn't fully understand. Trying to operate a system without understanding the program is foolish—like flying blind. When I used the wrong input commands, I created the equivalent of disease in the computer and erased the disk. Trying to operate your body without understanding its design is also like flying blind. Many errors are based on insufficient information as to how to operate our human system. We often input unhealthy things, creating dis-ease.

Problems also exist because of the level of noise in our environment. Noise is analogous to the static in any machine or computer system. Noise is confused or confusing information from any source, internal or external. Noise is unhelpful, unwanted meaning! Noise is the chatter in your head, the memory tapes that get stuck and play the same tune again and again. Noise might be the memory of a daily admonition from your mother, the reprimand from a teacher, or the tease from a classmate.

Noise in the human mind comes from your biases, belief systems, unhealthy seedthoughts, past experiences and memory. Noise distorts the messages you receive. To the extent that you are unaware of your biases, internal noise will color your perception of reality. Optimal health requires accurate information about what you feel and need. Distortion is the inability to perceive the true meaning of a new event or sensation.

Intrapersonal Communication

When mind, body, and emotions are unified, each part of the system receives accurate communication. If a mind/body dichotomy prevails, error and distortion is more likely. If you are experiencing ill health, there may be a lack of clear and effective communication *from your body to your mind*. Ill health also signals that communication *from your mind to your body* probably contains unhealthy messages. This static in your intra-personal communication—you with yourself—can lead to illness.

In an article in *Smithsonian* titled "A Molecular Code Links Emotions, Mind And Health," Stephen S. Hall wrote, "The classic view of the body as three separate systems is challenged as research points the way to the new medicine of the 21st century....Some biologists believe we need to rethink some long-cherished principles, beginning with medicine's traditional separation of the central nervous system (the seat of thought, memory and emotion) from the endocrine system (which secretes powerful hormones) and the immune system (which defends the body from microbial invasions.)"[116]

Molecules carry messages amongst the various anatomical systems. These powerful biochemicals, called neurotransmitters or hormones, have been referred to as "informational substances" by M.I.T. neuroscientist Francis O. Schmitt. Some researchers say that learning how and why these substances work may influence medicine in the future similarly to the way genetic code research influenced medicine in the past. Further quoting Hall, "The informational substances, many of which are known to have a powerful effect on mood and emotion, provide a molecular way to understand the long-suspected connection between state of mind and state of health."[117]

Schmitt's biochemical information substances seem to be the vehicles that carry messages—thoughts and emotions—to cells throughout the body. These messengers then stimulate the production of other substances that enhance or detract from the body's functions. The mind, body, and emotions intersect in the immune system, which affects your ability to ward off disease.

Anything in the nature of static in your system, whether physical or mental in origin, can produce unhelpful biochemical information. This pollution renders other systems less effective for the job they were meant to do.

Interpersonal Communication

Other people's words can contribute to the noise that prevents you from knowing what is really true for you. A message from someone you love, trust and respect can distort your own perception of reality. Someone else's ideas, even someone you don't like, might lead you to misperceptions and faulty conclusions.

From the children's game of "telephone," we learn how secondhand communication changes the original message. Hearsay is not accepted in most courts of law because secondhand, the original meaning is so often distorted. Putting credence in such noise can mislead and cause dis-ease in individuals as well as relationship problems.

Static in interpersonal communication—you with others—can lead to unhappy personal relationships. If you aren't getting along with someone, there is probably some miscommunication, or distortion of meaning. Distortion results in misunderstanding and a breakdown in communication between individuals, families, and nations. Clear communication is always necessary for harmony.

Words often mean different things to different people. For example, take the word "upset." What do you mean when you say, "I am upset"? To some, "upset" means you are angry; to others, it means afraid; while to others, "upset" might indicate sadness. To complicate matters further, "I am upset" is a statement that might mean different things to you at different times. Now observe a sample dialogue to see how distorted communication can occur.

- Mary says to John: "I feel really upset (meaning sad)."
- John hears, "Oh, she's upset (meaning angry) with me. What did I do?"

- John responds angrily: "What's wrong with you? What did I do to hurt you?
- Mary is flabbergasted. Why is John acting angry towards her when she is already so upset? Mary hasn't yet realized that John thinks she is angry at him.
- Mary replies angrily: "I can't see why you're yelling at me when I feel so upset."
- John then goes on to justify his outburst and the two of them move further and further apart.

These kinds of communication difficulties occur quite often, causing untold personal misery and damage to what might otherwise be good relationships.

Body Messages

Just as redundancy is built into this book for purposes of clarity, redundancy is part of the body's communication. Messages are repeated often, especially when they are ignored or misunderstood. Your body will speak louder and more clearly, until you get it.

For example, if I become accustomed to experiencing a dull ache in my lower back, I might come to accept it as inevitable. I may ignore it and not do anything about it. Thereafter, a dull ache in my lower back ceases to transmit any new information to me, information which might be useful for improving my state of health. Instead a louder message, perhaps intense sharp pain, would be necessary before I would take action. For me back pain leads me to visit my chiropractor, have a massage, or take a bath in my Jacuzzi. Now that I am more aware of my body's messages, I am quick to listen to my body and take appropriate action.

My friend Anne, who has been quite overweight for many years, developed a kidney stone. After passing the stone she talked to me about her weight. She said, "I've been waiting (weighting) for something to happen, some illness. I knew if I stayed fat something bad would happen to my body." Fear of suffering can be a potent motivating force. Anne's painful experience was her incentive to start exercising and change her diet. Eventually she lost quite a bit of weight. Then one day someone, who meant no harm, said "Anne, you are so thin."

Months later, after regaining some weight, she recognized that "you are so thin" was the seedthought which triggered her several month's eating binge. She said, "those words remind me of my parents who often told me 'eat—you are so thin.'" Apparently her family had at some point been concerned that she would be undernourished. The "eat" programming remained long after it ceased to serve her. Fortunately, recognizing the trigger for her eating binge has enabled her to interrupt the process and erase the "so thin" programming.

Body weight messages are frequently ignored. Too much weight is often caused by eating too much of the wrong food. Also, eating too little of the right foods results in undernourishnment and the need for more food. The first message signaling poor eating habits might be feelings of tiredness, or an unsightly body. Our bodies usually signal us in the most benign ways possible. Ignoring the body's first weight message may result in more physical discomforts. The messages then get louder and clearer until they can no longer be ignored. High blood pressure, heart disease, liver and gall bladder troubles, and many more symptoms are often, though not always, related to improper eating habits.

Many years ago, long before I knew anything about natural healing, I would suffer bouts of intense headache pain on and off for weeks at a time. I was mis-diagnosed as having "sinus headaches" and spent years of time and money on ineffective treatments. Later I received the accurate label of "cluster-migraine" but had no clue as to the cause. Potent medicine eased the pain. Then I lost my voice so I quit smoking, thinking cigarettes were the cause of my laryngitis. Quitting smoking had an unexpected benefit for me. I stopped having the migraine headaches. Years later I read that allergies to nicotine, alcohol, and other addictive substances can cause migraine headaches.

The cause of my headaches had been obscured by my incomplete information. I wasn't sensitive enough to discern the harmful effects smoking was having on my body. Now my awareness of my body—my language connection—has strengthened significantly. My mind/body communication gets clearer and smarter all the time. After I quit smoking in 1970, I literally felt a pain in my chest any time I even thought of inhaling a cigarette of any kind.

Technological Feedback

Highly sensitive medical technology is available to give you accurate biological feedback. This helps when you are unclear about the cause of a specific sensation or symptom. Most things that help you to know yourself better are very useful, and medical technology is no exception. Tools such as cardiograms, stress tests, X rays, Nuclear, Bone, MRI and CT scans, plus sophisticated chemical analysis of blood, hair, and urine can give you much-needed information. This diagnostic technology can catch potential breakdowns in your system even before sickness makes you feel ill. Include in your Operating Manual these and other diagnostic techniques to be used when appropriate. Help your body to overcome the dis-easing effects of noise in the mind/body system by periodic preventive maintenance in the form of regular medical checkups.

But the key to good health is static-free, accurate, intrapersonal communication: you with yourself, and your mind with your body. Just as peeling away the layers of an onion's skin releases its essence, you develop clear inner vision and intuition by uncovering your unconscious beliefs. Increasing numbers of doctors are open to a variety of healing modalities and will often assist you in finding the way. Static-free self-communication is available to anyone willing to invest time and energy in the process.

It is often useful to take a continuing education course, self-help workshop, meditation class or to work with a private coach or counselor to guide you towards effective self-understanding. Some resources are listed in the Appendix of this book. The purpose of such work is to de-stress, which always improves your internal communication. It also helps you to transform and improve the quality of your life. Participants often report major breakthroughs in many areas of their lives.

Sometimes it's useful to go on retreat and immerse yourself in an intensive program to get to know yourself better. The Kripalu Center for Yoga and Health in Massachusetts is one such highly regarded place that has been around for a long time. Kripalu offers many programs designed to improve your well-being. One 14-day residential program called "Kripalu Health for Life" combines many of the elements that promote good health: good diet and nutrition; exercise; bodywork; relaxation and meditation training; plus hours of experiential workshops which enhance self-awareness. The program includes physician and R.N. supervision and on-going support services where possible.

Kripalu reported the following documented results:

- **Hypertension**—80% of those using medication prior to the program significantly reduced or eliminated their need for medication;

- **Cholesterol**—those with above normal levels achieved an average 15% decrease;

- **Triglycerides**—average drop 15%;

- **Diabetes**—all participants with adult-onset diabetes decreased or eliminated their need for medication;

- **Weight**—average loss 8 pounds for those desiring to lose weight.[118]

The Truth Process

The *truth process* is an important technique to include in your Operating Manual. When you can objectively observe yourself and then truthfully describe to yourself what you are feeling, you will know yourself better. I first recognized this in 1973 during *est,* a weekend training program. Though this particular program is no longer available, it has spawned many others that use similar techniques. This workshop was about finding the truth about the way *it* (life) is for us at any given moment in time. During *the truth process*, a guided exercise, we practiced telling the truth about what we were really experiencing, instead of fooling ourselves with excuses and illusions. I still use this process. It is effective in relieving pain among other feelings and can be used in conjunction with medication and other therapies.

If I have a headache, I stop what I am doing and observe the headache carefully, exploring what I am experiencing. I stay emotionally detached and describe the shape, color, and temperature of the sensations I feel in my head. It helps to have someone ask me questions about those qualities. Some people feel silly doing this, but it is a very effective technique, especially with children. I then notice any meaning I attach to the physical sensations I label "headache," looking for reasons to explain what I am experiencing.

I scan my memory banks for all the causes I have ever associated with headache, such as allergy, not enough sleep, or too much sun. Discovering the cause can help prevent future headaches. Now that I no longer smoke and I eat more carefully, I am relatively headache-free. When I do have a headache, my body has sent an effective warning signal, communicated to me through pain, that some change is in order. I usually get the message!

During the *est* training, each trainee selected a problem to focus on. While thinking about the condition which we hoped to eliminate—perhaps a physical sensation like a headache or an emotion such as jealousy—we described to ourselves the physical sensations and emotions that we were feeling. We noted the thoughts we were thinking. Doing this process taught me to objectively witness myself. An objective witness doesn't get sucked in by the lies of the mind.

Afterwards, many trainees talked about the releases that they achieved during the truth process. It seems that by minutely observing and describing their experience at that moment, they caused the sensations, emotions, and the experience itself to vanish. I am not sure why observing a painful condition makes it disappear. The explanation given us by the trainer was "When you fully experience your experience it will disappear." To me that meant that *we are supposed to learn something from each of our experiences, and when we do, we can move on to the next experience.* By objectively observing ourselves we extract the necessary information in order to learn from whatever happens in our lives.

Ultimately the self-attention of objectively witnessing yourself will expand your understanding of each event in your life and the effects of these events on you. Understanding leads to increased awareness of how you need to act to care for your human instrument to achieve a better quality of life.

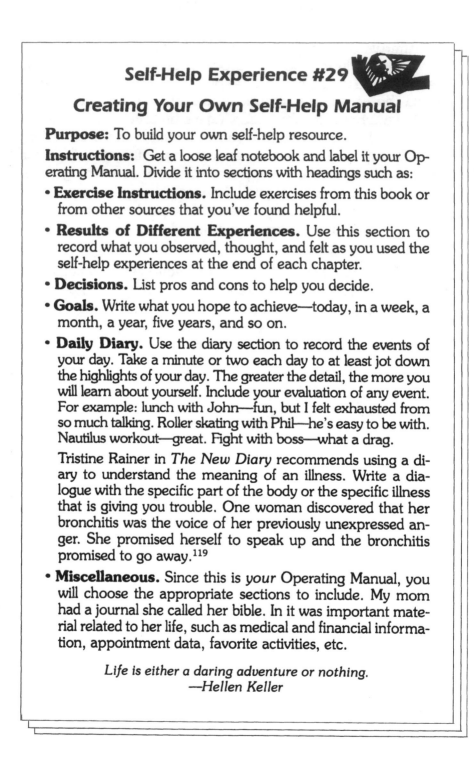

Self-Help Experience #29

Creating Your Own Self-Help Manual

Purpose: To build your own self-help resource.

Instructions: Get a loose leaf notebook and label it your Operating Manual. Divide it into sections with headings such as:

- **Exercise Instructions.** Include exercises from this book or from other sources that you've found helpful.

- **Results of Different Experiences.** Use this section to record what you observed, thought, and felt as you used the self-help experiences at the end of each chapter.

- **Decisions.** List pros and cons to help you decide.

- **Goals.** Write what you hope to achieve—today, in a week, a month, a year, five years, and so on.

- **Daily Diary.** Use the diary section to record the events of your day. Take a minute or two each day to at least jot down the highlights of your day. The greater the detail, the more you will learn about yourself. Include your evaluation of any event. For example: lunch with John—fun, but I felt exhausted from so much talking. Roller skating with Phil—he's easy to be with. Nautilus workout—great. Fight with boss—what a drag.

  Tristine Rainer in *The New Diary* recommends using a diary to understand the meaning of an illness. Write a dialogue with the specific part of the body or the specific illness that is giving you trouble. One woman discovered that her bronchitis was the voice of her previously unexpressed anger. She promised herself to speak up and the bronchitis promised to go away.[119]

- **Miscellaneous.** Since this is *your* Operating Manual, you will choose the appropriate sections to include. My mom had a journal she called her bible. In it was important material related to her life, such as medical and financial information, appointment data, favorite activities, etc.

Life is either a daring adventure or nothing.
—Hellen Keller

Self-Help Experience #30

Understanding Pain Messages

Purpose: To improve your general level of health. The body is as logical as a computer; what you program in is what you get. The design function of pain is to make you aware of a malfunction which has the potential of making your system inoperative. When you first experience a pain, you need to stop and ask yourself some questions.

Instructions:

1. *What does the pain mean?* The answer to this question will lead you to the appropriate treatment. Don't panic. Clear decoding of body signals is essential. For example, if you experience chest pain, there are many possible explanations. Check the meaning of the message by noticing any accompanying body messages. Are you nauseous? sweating? short of breath? Does the pain radiate? Does your heart palpitate? If you have these symptoms and are over a certain age, you might label your pain as heart attack.

   If accompanying your pain in the chest you are having chills, fever, symptoms of cold and flu, you might suspect pneumonia. Chest pains can also be caused by a broken rib, by a burst air sac in the lung, indigestion, gallstones, pulled muscles, or other factors.

2. *What have I been doing: to or with my body?* Your body tells you through sensation if you are acting inappropriately. If your hand starts to feel too hot, you're too close to the fire. Are you eating right, too much, too little, healthy foods? Exercising enough, or too much? Are you spending quiet time with yourself? What kinds of thoughts have been dwelling in your mind?

3. *What actions do I need to take to relieve these symptoms and improve my body?* Sit quietly for a few minutes and reflect on your answers to the above questions. Then

(continued) next page

the answer to this question will flow from the information you've received. You will know what to do or who to see to guide you into appropriate treatment.

4. *Take action.* Use the pain message to improve the quality of your life by acting on what you've learned. For example: I discovered some food allergies were causing me to itch so I stopped eating those foods. If you think you have pneumonia, see a doctor, and follow his instructions. If you have frequent headaches and recognize a cause, eliminate that cause from your life. Act on what you learn from any discomfort you experience. Get the message!

Belief is a potent medicine.
—Steven E. Locke and Douglas Colligan

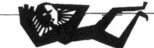

Self-Help Experience #31

The Truth Process

Purpose: To discover truth and relieve pain. To release unwanted behavior patterns such as jealousy, insecurity or procrastination.

Sue, the woman we met in an earlier chapter recognized her seedthought, "I don't want to hear that," during the truth process and freed herself of recurrent ear infections. This nonjudgmental witnessing can be used to ease any pain, whether physical or emotional in origin.

With physical pain, first do exercise #30 to understand any pain messages. You might be resisting the pain by tensing your body, thus making matters worse. Your physical sensations will probably change during this process before the pain leaves completely. Your focused attention can cause the pain to intensify momentarily but it will usually ease quickly.

Instructions:

1. When you are experiencing pain, stop what you are doing and objectively, without judgment, observe the pain. Don't ignore it. Experience it completely. If you are using this process to release an emotion or change an unwanted behavior pattern, begin by thinking about the behavior.

2. Notice your state of mind and emotions related to the sensations you are feeling and the thoughts you are thinking. Are you angry, sad, frustrated, etc.?

3. Stay emotionally detached as you describe the shape, color, and temperature of any sensations you feel. It helps to have someone ask you questions about those qualities. Pretend your pain or emotion has a color and a shape.

4. What meaning do you attach to your physical sensations? Scan your memory banks for past causes of similar sensations. What reasons explain or justify your pain?

5. Is there any situation in your present life that might be contributing to this current pain or upset?

6. Recall any earlier, similar situations related to the one you are now experiencing.

7. Go through these steps 1–6 a second time.

8. Thank your body and your mind for what the discomfort is teaching you.

9. Acknowledge any new truth you have learned. Write it in your Operating Manual or Journal. See Self-help Experience # 29 for instructions on creating your Operating Manual.

The healing process is made up of unconditional love,
forgiveness, and letting go of fear.
—Gerald Jampolsky

Self-Help Experience #32

Relaxation Activities

Purpose: To center yourself and clear mental distractions during an upset. Read through the following list of possibilities. Some may seem odd and not in keeping with your temperament. Try doing some you've never done before. Set time aside for some relaxation activities each day. Be open to new activities and new hobbies.

Instructions:

1. Walk barefoot on the beach or grass. This works even in cold weather.

2. Hug a tree. It may sound silly but try it anyway. Trees really are our friends, and their continuity of being is a valuable reminder of the central values at the core of life.

3. Read something you normally don't read.

4. Become a couch potato and vegetate for a time.

5. Attend a worship service with the religious group of your choice.

6. Read your Bible. If you don't have one, get one.

7. Listen to a guided meditation tape.

8. Play spiritual music. Anything from hymns to New Age music can induce relaxation.

9. Get up and dance to your favorite music.

10. Do some art work or any creative activity.

11. Do anything "just for the fun of it."

12. Fly a kite.

13. List your favorite relaxation activities in your Operating Manual.

14. Create a list of things to try in the future.

Laughter is a tranquilizer with no side effects.
—Arnold Glasow

When the going gets tough, the tough get going.

Count your blessings.

A stitch in time saves nine; know yourself.

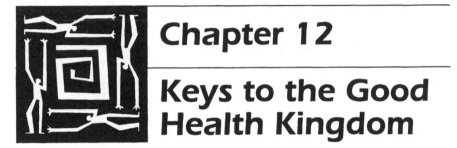

Chapter 12

Keys to the Good Health Kingdom

We each have an ongoing inner dialogue. A voice of judgment speaks to us continuously, analyzing and evaluating our experience. ("What voice?" you may ask. "The one that asked that question." I would answer.) Through introspection, a kind of meditation on oneself, one is able to process the plethora of signals one has to deal with each day, to make sense out of the complex stimuli in our internal and external environment.

Life works according to your ability to process information clearly, effectively, and meaningfully. A healthy, purposeful existence and rewarding relationships with others require practice in coding and decoding, as well as time for the practice to be effective. Through years of training, I have become expert at witnessing myself in a relatively objective way, and clearly describing what I experience, usually (but not always) without judging or condemning myself. It was this ability to witness myself that enabled me to write this book from a point of personal understanding. Witnessing myself and coming to grips with my own experience taught me empathy and compassion for others.

Intuition

Intuition, the direct knowledge or *awareness of something* without conscious attention or reasoning, will tell you when to see a doctor, when to get some exercise, when to rest. We all have some degree of intuition whether we pay attention to it or not. I know when I need a chiropractic adjustment, even if I can't describe any strong sensations. I feel something, and I have learned to interpret and trust what I feel. Perhaps people with reliable intuition know how to keep the message-distorting static out of their feedback system. Perhaps intuitive people have a strong language connection, fine-tuned by their ability to decode subtle body messages.

My daughter Jennifer has a well-developed intuitive sense. She often says, "I don't know why, but something tells me I should do this," or "A voice inside me tells me not to eat this." When she was younger she said the voice was separate from her (and maybe it was). But now she says it's a part of herself that she trusts.

Intuitively you can know what ails you long before it can be medically verified. A patient of Westport, Connecticut psychiatrist Harry Brown, M.D., had a dream about wanting to eat red meat and blood. Dr. Brown said, "She was distressed by her dream. I recommended she take a blood test, and we found she was anemic." She tapped her inner knowledge and dreamt a signal for her mind to act on. She was then guided by a skilled physician who became her partner in taking corrective action.

The mind/body/emotions represent a continuous, closed-circuit communication system with instantaneous feedback. Meditation provides a pathway to clearer self-communication, a way to reconnect the seemingly separate parts of your system and bring back health. Developing your intuition is a side benefit. Meditation involves experiencing a quieter mind, without the judgmental thoughts and memories that often intrude on your experience. During meditation you more easily recognize the messages coming from your body, your emotions, and your subconscious mind. You can eliminate the noisy interference of unproductive, unhealthy thoughts—freeing yourself from the distortions that cause disease.

Varieties of Meditation

In various meditation systems you are told: Sit with a straight spine or lie flat on your back with eyes closed. Observe your breath by focusing your attention on inhaling and exhaling. If you start thinking about something else, your attention has wandered from your breath. Don't think about the thoughts, just notice them, and return your awareness to your breath. Some teachers tell you to follow the path of your breath as it travels through your body. For me, that means to imagine where the air I breathe goes after entering my body.

Another meditation system involves the repetition of a mantra. A mantra is a syllable, word, or phrase with spiritual significance and special creative power. "Mantra" is a Sanskrit word meaning "a sound that frees." A mantra can either be repeated inwardly or chanted out loud. The focus on the word or phrase keeps the mind occupied.

Most religious traditions have well-known words appropriate for mantra meditation:

- the Jewish "Sh'ma Yisrael... Hear O Israel, the Lord is God the Lord is One"
- the Catholic "Hail Mary full of grace, the Lord is One"
- the Christian "Come Holy Spirit"
- the Islamic "Allah-u-Akbar—God is the Greatest"
- the Islamic "La Illaha Illa 'llah hu—There is no God but God"
- the Tibetan Buddhist "Om Mane Padme Om—Blessed is the jewel in the lotus."
- the Buddhist "Nam Myoho Renge Kyo," a chant asking for Buddha's enlightenment and to change one's karma
- the Hindu "Namaste" or "Jai Bhagwan" which means I bow to the Divine in you.

- the Hindu "Om Nama Shivaya," literally I bow to Lord Shiva; although some state it as "The God in me bows to the God in you" or even "Thy will, not mine, be done"
- the Hebrew prayer for healing "El Nah, R'fah Nah Lah" "O God pray, heal her"
- The Universal "Peace be with you"
- Hallelujah, Amen, Shalom, Maranatha, Aum or Om or even Abracadabra

Different teachers train or initiate people in the use of their favored tones, sounds, and words. One system I like includes chanting the vowels of the English alphabet and imagining a specific color with each vowel sound. Some people achieve good results just counting or repeating "one, two," bringing on the relaxation necessary for meditation.

In both the Jewish and Christian traditions, meditation is often part of prayer, worship and contemplation. Meditation may either make you more present and more aware (to know yourself better), or conversely, less present and less aware (to forget yourself and know God better). Each state is beneficial.

Quieting the mind by focusing pointedly on one thing, be it your breath, a specific prayer, or a mantra, takes practice. Daily sessions of at least twenty minutes are recommended. Because meditation is an active experience most teachers recommend meditating on an empty stomach so your energy won't be required for digestion. Steady use of these relaxing techniques eventually filters out the thoughts that prevent you from hearing and understanding your inner self.

Many claims have been made regarding the effectiveness of meditation. Long-time meditators often report that they feel more relaxed; need less sleep; think more clearly; and cope better with stress, among other claims. Many people who have experienced remission of a chronic or terminal disease note that meditation, in one form or another, was a key part of their healing program.

Researchers at the Medical Center of the University of California at Irvine found that the practice of Transcendental Meditation (TM) increased the flow of blood to the brain. "The average increase in blood flow in participants was 65% greater than that measured when the subject merely relaxed. This may account, at least in part, for the role of meditation in improved mental performance observed in earlier studies."[120]

Alcoholics use drink to cope with stress. A *Brain/Mind Bulletin* article reports that practicing meditation gives alcoholics another coping tool. Two Chicago doctors—alcoholism program treatment directors—emphasize that "these procedures must not be thought of as a form of treatment but as an adjunct to medical and psychiatric approaches during the period of acute withdrawal."[121]

Brain/Mind Bulletin also reports on the helpfulness of meditation in reducing alcoholic drinking in general, in heavy social drinkers. In one study of different relaxation therapies to support reduced drinking, meditation (Dr. Herbert Benson's relaxation response) was found to be the "best option for alcoholism treatment among several treatments evaluated.[122] Other options were progressive muscular relaxation and what was called "bibliotherapy," restful reading twice daily. A control group received no therapy at all. It seems that subjects taught to meditate were most likely to continue the relaxation program and thus achieved more lasting reduction in their alcohol consumption.

Meditation can help many conditions. Henry Reed, Virginia Beach psychologist and dream research authority, conducted a study with members of A.R.E.—The Association for Research and Enlightenment. It was discovered that meditation improves dream recall, at least in experienced meditators.[123] The New York Telephone Company adopted meditation as part of its regular health maintenance program after an eighteen-month study on stress reduction involving 154 employees.[124] Other experiments using meditation have demonstrated its value in reducing hypertension.[125]

A study of the effects of Transcendental Meditation on prisoners incarcerated in Folsom prison in California indicated significant enhancement in mental health. A three-month study of 26 prisoners and a control group of 30 other non-meditating prisoners examined anxiety, neuroticism, hostility, aggressive behavior, self-concept, resting blood pressure, and pulse rates. Pre-test and post-test smoking and sleep patterns also were studied for the meditating prisoners. After three months, the TM meditators were "less anxious, less prone to violence, more stable and had an improved self-concept."[126] After the study was completed, there was a waiting list of 500 prisoners wanting to be trained in the technique.

According to practitioners of Transcendental Meditation (TM), by meditating we can affect the thoughts, feelings and actions of others—even those who might not be meditating themselves. TM founder Maharishi Mahesh Yogi believes that TM meditation affects the consciousness of people in the immediate surroundings, the size of the area depending on the number of meditators.

Long time meditator David A. Tapper told me:

"Any experienced meditator, of whatever variety of meditation, has had the experience of feeling the charge in a room increase as more people assemble to meditate. The TM folk have studied the phenomenon, and have published their results in peer-evaluated publications.

"For example, several studies have been made in Atlanta, Georgia, where a large group of meditators meditated together for a several month period in one of the more crime infested areas of Atlanta. As the time period progressed, less crime was reported to the police in the area, and the number of emergency admissions to hospitals went down dramatically. Then the group was moved to another precinct. Lo and behold, the crime and violent accident rate in the new district went down, and those rates went up in the district which had been abandoned.

"TM experimenters also looked at this consciousness effect in Lebanon during the period of active hostilities. As a gauge of the effect they were having, an independent agency counted the headlines from the Lebanese and Israeli press on the number of violent incidents in Lebanon. As more meditators practiced the TM technique, there were fewer and fewer incidents. As the number of meditators fluctuated downward, there were more incidents.

"Maharishi's theory is that when the square root of one percent of a population of an area meditates a distinct peaceful effect will be felt by that population. The statistics bear that out. And I find it fascinating that statistical science bears out some mystical assumptions."[127]

Mindfulness

The Zen concept of meditation is mindfulness, in which you stay aware of your present reality without the distraction of extraneous thoughts. For example, when you are washing the dishes, you keep all your attention on washing the dishes, so that you fully experience washing the dishes. Since it's not possible to focus clearly on two thoughts at one time, worry tends to disappear during mindfulness. Stated simply, it means doing whatever you do with an attitude of total absorption. Mindfulness is a state of being fully in the moment.

Witnessing yourself is a form of mindfulness in which you focus inwardly on all you are experiencing at any given moment, including your thoughts and feelings. The witness, an objective observer, is *you watching you* without judgment. The idea is to detach yourself from your surroundings so that all attention is focused on your inner process. I often find this difficult. My mind wants to wander, think of other things, do its own activity. It takes effort and strong intention to control my mind.

Once during a meditation, I encountered a potent visual metaphor for the objective observer *observing* myself. Though my eyes were closed, a large blue eye appeared in my visual field. The eye (I) was watching me. The blue eye was the "I" of my Self, watching me even while I watched It.

If your mind continually dwells on a problem, writing it out in your journal is useful, as it saves the data without your constantly needing to re-play the mental tape.

These descriptions of mindfulness, insight, and witnessing are based on my own experience of the meaning of these terms and may not be the same as the meaning used by any specific group. When the mind is quieted by any means, you gain insight—that special sense of "seeing things as they really are." Your expanding awareness leads to more appropriate lifestyle choices.

All systems of meditation take practice, self-discipline, and an attitude of calm, centered acceptance of oneself. The rewards of each form of meditation are great, proportionate to the disciplined effort of the meditator, just like any other self-improvement activity. To meditate is to put into practice the desire to be increasingly in touch with your inner world. Meditation can be practiced in a variety of ways throughout the day.

Moving Meditations

Not all meditation practices are done sitting quietly. There are also moving meditations. Examples include Tai Chi, Hatha Yoga, and many of the martial arts. Of course, the movement alone is beneficial to the body. But in each of these systems, the mental focus on the activity results in a release of tension in mind and body.

My favorite activity for relaxation, meditation, and exercise is walking. During walking I solve problems, gain inspiration for writing, use affirmations, exercise my body, and reduce stress by releasing negative energy. I am in charge of my mind's activity during a walk. But if I am agitated about some real or imagined problem, my mind often takes charge and runs through its memory bank of tapes related to my problem. I allow this process to go on for a while because I learn about my unconscious feelings by observing my upsetting thoughts. I can then do what it takes to improve my situation.

Dancing is effective as social activity, for gaining fitness, de-stressing, and releasing emotion. Classical ballet, jazz, folk, and social dancing often require focused attention to perform them properly. Music helps us reach the non-conscious mind. Just listening to music often unlocks the door that seems to block feelings and thoughts, allowing images to arise spontaneously. Images are the door to the not-yet-conscious, and music is a key which unlocks it. Any physical activity where you are fully involved—with music or without—can become a method of meditation.

Prayer Heals

Personal prayer is another form of meditation which absorbs the mind. It can be practiced sitting in stillness or moving around. Use your own words or verses from Sacred Texts such as the Torah, Bible, Koran and so on. The Lord's Prayer and the Twenty-Third Psalm have brought me comfort. The Gayatri Mantra and the World Invocation are other ways to use a prayer-focused mind to achieve a specific result in the world. One of my favorite non-sectarian prayers is the *Serenity Prayer*: "God grant me the serenity to accept the things I cannot change, the will and courage to change the things I can, and the wisdom to know the difference."

Prayer is effective whether you pray for yourself or if others pray for you. People will often pray for strangers and celebrities, as well as for loved ones in dire straits. In the nationally reported case of the jogger brutally attacked in New York's Central Park, thousands, maybe millions of people prayed for her recovery, which has gone beyond the expectations of her doctors. In another case, the whole world waited for toddler Jessica McClure to be rescued from the well in Texas. Then too, our prayers were answered. Elizabeth Taylor returned home just a week after brain surgery to remove a tumor. Perhaps the prayers of Taylor's millions of fans really did have an extra positive effect.

A belief in God or a Higher Power is a core belief for a majority of Americans. According to a Newsweek magazine poll "Most Americans say prayers every day, even though no one knows why only some are answered."[128] We seem to believe that there is something beyond ourselves that will act in our behalf for our highest good. Furthermore, most people intuitively understand that their words have power and that somehow the words of a prayer will work: "87% say that God answers prayers."[129]

We use words and thoughts in our attempts to influence this Source of all healing, just as in other parts of our everyday life we use words and thoughts that influence and control our body. Whenever people use words to speak with God, they are simultaneously planting positive seedthoughts within themselves. (According to the concepts in this book, prayer is also a healing conversation, another aspect of the language connection.)

Citing numerous studies of the efficacy of prayer in healing, Larry Dossey, M.D., writes, "The evidence is overwhelming that prayer functions at a distance to change physical processes in a variety of organisms, from bacteria to humans."[130] Some would say that the primary value in praying for the well-being of another is in the effect that it has on the one doing the praying. I would partly agree. When I pray for someone else, it does help me to feel better, a good reason to pray for others. But I feel certain that my prayers for others reach and affect them as well in ways I may never understand. Dr. Dossey's book *Healing Words* confirms my belief in the effect of personal prayers.

A double-blind randomized study by cardiologist Randy Byrd using 393 coronary care unit patients at San Francisco General Hospital adds weight to the belief that patients have fewer medical complications when prayed for. 192 patients were prayed for and 201 were not. Neither patients nor Dr. Byrd were aware of who was being prayed for until the data was recorded. The people praying were told the patients' first names and diagnoses. Byrd had recruited "born again" Christians from home prayer groups to pray daily for several patients each, using whatever prayer they chose. Statistics showed the two groups of patients were equally sick when they entered the hospital, but that patients who were prayed for had fewer complications during their stay.[131] Dr. Dossey commented "even some hard-boiled skeptics agreed on the significance of Byrd's findings..." After acknowledging that it sounds like this study will stand up to scrutiny one of these skeptics said "Maybe we doctors ought to be writing on our order sheets, 'pray three times a day.' If it works, it works."[132]

Dr. Jacqueline Ruzga, a Fairfield, Connecticut chiropractor has an interesting prayer ritual which helps prepare her to see patients. She told me: "I go into each of my exam rooms and touch the exam table and say to myself, 'Please God make my patients healthy. Make sure I do the right adjustment on each one of them.'"[133]

Judy Chessin, a clinical nursing specialist in geriatric psychiatry, is an instructor at Yale University School of Nursing and at times a hospice nurse. Speaking on a panel of medical professionals who were discussing the role of prayer and spirituality in caring for their patients, she said, "I practice in a holistic way. That means striving to meet whatever needs my individual patients may have. I will help them articulate their needs by listening carefully, for what they don't say, as well as what they do say. At times my patients need help in communicating to their family and expressing their feelings. I might give a patient a hug, hold their hand, or pray with them. Although I am Jewish, I learned to say the Rosary because one of my Alzheimer patients couldn't remember all the words. Saying the Rosary prayer was important to him and seemed to reduce his depression and anxiety bringing him peace and joy."[134]

How You Can Use These Tools

An important key to a healthy, happy life is the willingness to spend some quiet time with yourself each day. A daily period of solitude allows you to communicate with yourself while your mind recharges its batteries. Include such time in your personal Operating Manual. Then you will be better able to cope with the normal—and not so normal—stresses and strains of everyday life. A healthy, purposeful existence and rewarding relationships with others will be the result.

During chanting, meditation or prayer, as you unify your mind/body/emotions and reconnect your seemingly separate parts, you expand your ability to choose freely and to process information clearly, effectively, and meaningfully. Clearer mind/body communication means you will know yourself better. You will begin to recognize and accept your emotions, uncover harmful beliefs and Seedthoughts, and begin to change them through the power of creative thinking. Joyfully accept it! An attitude of gratitude is a primary ingredient for a happy, healthy, peaceful, fulfilled life.

Self-Help Experience #33

Mindfulness Meditation

Purpose: To practice witnessing yourself without judgment.

Instructions:

Practice each one of the four categories below by itself for a few sessions of ten minutes each, until you gain proficiency in the technique. Sit straight with eyes closed. Later, after combining all the categories to practice the complete meditation, you will be able to effectively witness yourself throughout the day, even with your eyes open.

1. *Sensations from inside your physical body.* Focus attention on your physical body, watching your breath rise and fall. Note posture, physical attributes, and body sensations such as:

Taste
Temperature
Muscular tension
Color or lack of color behind your eyelids
Hunger pangs
Pain
Breath rate or ease of breathing

Sounds from the body such as stomach grumbling

Note whether the sensation is pleasant, unpleasant, or neutral. Because the mind works by classifying, you observe your mind classifying. You may realize that thoughts have a creative life of their own.

2. Sensations from outside your body. Note sensations arising external to your body, such as:
The feel of air moving across your body.
The touch of the object you are sitting on.
The air temperature where you are sitting.
The kinds of sounds you hear. Is it quiet, noisy, calming, distracting?
Is your sitting space brightly lit or darkened?
Does the space feel cramped or roomy?

Note whether the sensation associated with each item is pleasant, unpleasant, or neutral.

3. Your state of mind. Note your state of mind and how it shifts. Are you annoyed, impatient, at peace? Each time a new state appears, note "mind impatient," "mind peaceful," "mind doubting," or even "mind eager."

4. Visual pictures and memories. Note any visual pictures or memories that come to mind. Notice how you classify thoughts and evaluate them. There will be some overlapping of categories when you begin to practice, but that is fine because ultimately you will incorporate all the categories into a combined practice.

5. Combined practice. After practicing each of the four categories singly for several sitting sessions, you will be ready for combined practice. Plan to sit about 40 minutes. Your basic focus is on the breath. As you sit, observing your breath and posture, be ready to receive other impressions. Whatever you experience is to be noted, be it sensation, thought, feeling, or state of mind. When you have no other thoughts or experiences, when no other mindfulness category is operating, return to observing your breath.

(continued) next page

Eventually mindfulness will become your usual state. This monitoring may be difficult, even uncomfortable, but the results are remarkable, according to Justin Stone, from whose book *Meditation For Healing* this exercise is adapted. "For the first time we see how we actually operate; for the first time we have self-knowledge."[135] The mental delusions we subject ourselves to can disappear, healing sickness in the mind.

Trust your hunches. They're usually based on facts filed away just below the conscious level.
—Dr. Joyce Brothers

Self-Help Experience #34

A Ten-Step Plan to Improve Your Life

Purpose: A daily routine that will improve the quality of your life. Gandhi is reported to have said, "Total effort, total victory."

Instructions:

1. Keep a journal of your feelings every day.

2. Join a support group that meets at least once a month. Every week is better if you are in crisis or ill.

3. Live an hour at a time.

4. Meditate, pray, or listen to music at least once or twice a day.

5. Do some form of physical exercise each day.

6. Eat what you believe is a good diet.

7. While looking in the mirror, repeat aloud, "I love you (add your name)." Occasionally do this in front of a mirror while naked. Notice any negative judgments you have about yourself and cancel them.

8. Give thanks to a higher power for the good in your life.

Give thanks, too, for the trials you face. Learn something from them.

9. Hug at least one person every day.

10. Tell at least one person every day that you love them.

I don't think of all the misery, but of all the
beauty that still remains.
—Anne Frank

Self-Help Experience #35

Personal Prayers

Purpose: To connect you with a higher power.

Instructions: If you think you don't know how to pray, relax! It's just like talking to someone you love and trust, in your own words, in silence or aloud, wherever you happen to be—sitting, standing, walking, lying down, or even driving. Prayer is real and potent and comes from your heart when *you* choose the words. This is one of my favorite prayers for guidance and protection:

"Mother-Father-God, just now I ask for your presence, through the light of the Torah (or Christ or Allah etc.) and the Holy Spirit. Please fill, surround, and protect me with your radiant light. I give thanks for all that I have received. (Sometimes I give thanks for specific things.) I ask that only that which is for my highest good and the highest good of all will occur. Thank you! I ask that the light and the Holy Spirit be sent to (names of family members, friends, business associates, and world situations)."

The *National Center for Jewish Healing* shared this Healing Prayer from Rabbi Jim Michaels.

In my illness, Lord, I turn to you, for I am your creation.

(continued) next page

Your strength and courage are in my spirit,
and your powers of healing are within my body.
May it be your will to restore me to health.
In my illness I have learned what is great and what is small.
I know how dependent I am upon you.
My own pain and anxiety have been my teachers.
May I never forget this precious knowledge when I am well
  again.
Heal me, Lord and I shall be healed, save me and I shall be
  saved.
Comfort me, Lord, and shelter me in your love.
Blessed are you, Lord, the Faithful and merciful Healer. Amen.

From your lips to God's ear.
—Jewish Proverb

Self-Help Experience #36

Who's Responsible for Me?

Purpose: To accept personal responsibility for your life without condemning or judging yourself.

Instructions: *Remind yourself daily until these ideas become second nature:*

• I am responsible for my life.

• I choose what to think and feel.

• Responsibility does not imply blame, shame, or a negative evaluation of myself.

• Responsibility is my acceptance (without judgment) of the control I do have over my life.

• If not me, who?

• If not now, when?

Pain is inevitable, suffering is optional.
—Author Unknown

Self-Help Experience #37

Chanting Exercises

Purpose: Relaxation; quieting the mind; using sound creatively.

Instructions:

1. Have a reverent attitude before you begin to chant.

2. Some people sit cross-legged, others kneel, some sit in a chair and others choose to stand.

3. You can chant any of the mantras mentioned in this book, aloud or silently. Some teachers believe you must chant aloud, at least part of the time. The sound then vibrates and the vibration produces the result. Following are three chants I've used successfully, plus some others that are suitable:

- **Sh'ma Yisrael Adonai Eloheinu Adonai Echad.** Hear O Israel The Lord Is God The Lord Is One.

- **Om Namah Shivaya**—I surrender to God —Thy Will Not Mine Be Done.

- **Marantha**—Come Lord and Baruch Hashem—Praise God.

- **Hail Mary Full Of Grace The Lord Is One.**

- **Allah-u-Akbar**—God is Greater.

- **Om Mané Padmé Aum**—Blessed Is The Jewel In The Lotus.

- **Halleluyah, Shalom, Amen, Abracadabra**—Peace be with You.

- **Aum** or **Om**.

- Or even, **one/two/** one/two.

4. One system uses chanting a sound and visualizing a color together. When you chant a specific sound you think of a specific color. This requires a great deal of self-discipline and concentration. Chant the sounds *Om Ta Ma Ra Om* and think of a specific color with each sound.

(continued) next page

- When you chant **Om**, think **white**.
- When you chant **Ta**, think **red**.
- When you chant **Ma**, think **blue**.
- When you chant **Ra**, think **yellow**.

Chanting Your Own Affirmation. Recently during an MRI test to make sure my brain tumor had not recurred, I found that the banging noise of the test equipment made it difficult to chant, meditate or pray. So, I used an affirmation in step with the noisy rhythmic beat of the test, to chant inwardly. I repeated over and over, "Relaxed and happy from head to toe," saying one word for each beat. This allowed me to focus my mind and keep calm. Inwardly repeating my affirmative seedthought prevented me from thinking, "I can't stand this," "I hate this," "I am so scared," "This test is driving me crazy"—thoughts which I knew lurked beneath the surface of my mind. I felt great when the test was completed. The tumor is gone!

Meditation is not a means to an end. It is both
the means and the end.
—J. Krishnamurti

Self-Help Experience #38

The Breath Prayer

Purpose: To develop your own prayer.

Thanks to Rev. Rolland French, Jr; for sharing the Breath Prayer, from, *The Breath of Life*, by Ron DelBene, an Episcopal Priest. In the book he describes how one may develop one's own ritual prayer:

Instructions:

1. Sit in a comfortable position. Close your eyes, and remind yourself that God loves you and that you are in God's loving presence.

2. Recall a passage from scripture that puts you in a prayerful frame of mind. Consider " The Lord is my Shepherd" [Psalm 23] or "Be still, and Know that I am God!" [Psalm 46:10]

3. With your eyes closed, imagine that God is calling you by name. Hear God asking: "(your name), what do you want?

4. Answer God with whatever comes directly from your heart. Your answer might be a single word, such as "peace" or "love" or "forgiveness". Your answer could instead be a phrase or brief sentence, such as "I want to feel your forgiveness," or "I want to know your love."

5. Choose your favorite name for God. Choices commonly made include God, Jesus, Creator, Teacher, Light, Lord, Spirit, Shepherd, Adonai or Allah.

Combine your name for God with your answer to God's question" What do you want?" You then have your prayer. For example:

What I Want	Name for God	Possible Prayer
Peace	God	*Let me know your*
	peace, O God	
Love	Jesus	*Jesus, let me feel*
	your love.	
Rest	Shepherd	*My Shepherd, let me*
	rest in thee.	
Purpose	Adonai	Adonai, show me your
	purpose for my life.	

Pray with careful attention to breathing in and breathing out.[136]

I can see in what you call the dark, but which to me is golden.
I can see a God-made world, not a man-made world.
—Helen Keller

Self-Help Experience #39

Prayers to Memorize for Stressful Times

Purpose: to provide a distraction from harmful thoughts during times of stress.

Instructions: Prior to brain surgery, I memorized several longer prayers for use during tough times when I needed to keep my mind fully occupied. I used: *Psalm 23*, "The Lord is my Shepherd" and the *Lord's Prayer*, "Our Father who art in Heaven."

Following is an oft-repeated Islamic prayer and an English translation, courtesy of Imam Nasif Muhammad of Mosjia Al Aziz Temple in Bridgeport CT:

Al Faatiha

1. Bismillah Ir Rahmaan Ir Raheem
2. Al Hamdu lillaahi Rabbil 'Alameen
3. Ar Rahmaan Ir Raheem
4. Maaliki yaumid deen
5. Iyyaaka na'abudu wa iyyaaka nasta'een
6. Ihdinaa Siraatal Mustaqeen
7. Siraatal ladheena 'an amta alayhim

   Ghayril maghduubi alayhim wa lad dhaleen—Ameen

Translation: *The Opening*

1. With Allah's Name, The Merciful Benefactor, The Merciful Redeemer
2. All Praise be to Allah, the Lord of the Systems of Knowledge;
3. The Merciful Benefactor, the Merciful Redeemer
4. Master of the Day of Judgement
5. Thee do we worship, and Thine aid we seek.
6. Show us the Straight way,

7. The Way of those on whom Thou hast bestowed Thy Grace,
Those whose portion is not wrath, and go not astray.—
Amen

These next four expressions are used to remember Allah:

• **Allahu Akbar** = God is the Greatest

• **Subha-nallah** = Glory to God

• **Al Hamdu lillah** = All praise is due to God

• **La-ilaha illa-llah** = There is no deity but God

The following Hebrew prayer can be used when a loved one is ill; or one can use it to quiet the mind in general. This simple healing prayer is from numbers 12:13. **"El Nah, R'fah Nah Lah; O God Pray, Heal her."**

These were the Hebrew words spoken by Moses when he asked God to heal his sister Miriam. She had a skin eruption of snow-white scales at one time thought to be leprosy, but now often considered to be akin to psoriasis. It is the first healing prayer in the Bible. Generically one could translate El Nah, R'fah Nah Lah as "Please Heal (*insert name*)"

Our spiritual lives are strengthened as we find that precious balance between expectant trust in our higher power and responsible reliance on ourselves.
—Sefra Pitzele

Expect the best; be prepared for the worst.

Every day, in every way, I am getting better and better.

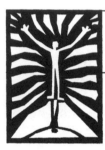

Chapter 13

Healing Techniques

An oft-studied research question in psycho-neuro-immunology is whether people can voluntarily change the function of their immune systems. A review of 22 studies suggests that self-regulation techniques can work. The studies used a variety of techniques including relaxation, imagery with and without music, self-hypnosis, meditation, and/or biofeedback. Of the 22 studies, 18 demonstrated changes on some immune measures following the use of one or more of the self-regulation techniques.[137] The following information will help you incorporate imagery techniques into your Operating Manual.

Picturing What You Want

In a guided meditation you follow a series of instructions during which you actively use your creative imagination. Guided meditations are useful when you know what is needed in order to heal yourself and can imagine that effect. For example, you might imagine: more antibodies to release a virus; a tumor getting smaller each day; you becoming slimmer; you swimming rather than smoking; etc. The use of mental imagery rests on the basic assumption that through our minds we can affect our bodies. Simply demonstrated, this is the principle behind thinking about tasting sweet chocolate and discovering that you salivate as a result of the thought, just as if the real chocolate had been thrust into your mouth.

Visualization is often part of a guided meditation. After quieting the mind using any of several techniques, the now-relaxed meditator imagines a specific result. Some people are good at visualizing and see clear images. Others sense or feel the desired change in different parts of the body. Some may hear or think words to guide the creative force within them. It's possible to achieve most goals with visualization. Corporate planners relate the value of visualization to ideas like management by objectives, targeting and goal setting.

Since visualization can be used to produce almost any desired result, it's a great aid in achieving your goals. Brian Boitano, upon winning the 1988 Olympic Gold Medal for figure skating said, "It was my dream performance that I'd visualized a million times, at least once a day, since I was nine years old."

My friend Nancy Nehlsen, co-author of *Princess Marjabelle Visits Lollygag Lake*, a picture book which teaches children good manners, taught her young son Alex visualization. She said:

"When Alex was in Little League I taught him how to practice hitting by pretending in his mind. I told him to imagine the end result before he got up to bat. The second time he tried this he got a single. He told me, 'I only imagined myself at first base.' In that game, on his third at-bat he got a triple. From then on, just before it was his turn to bat, he'd bow his head and visualize hitting well. Alex improved so much that the other moms at Little League have now all adopted my approach and taught their children this technique."[138]

Mental imagery for medical purposes has been used increasingly in recent years. Kenneth Pope of the Brentwood, California Veterans Administration Hospital, speaking at the first annual conference devoted to mental imagery said, "Mental imagery of blood vessels increasing in diameter, in combination with general relaxation, helps hypertensive patients lower their blood pressure. Those using relaxation alone were less effective."[139] He went on to explain that verbal language was limited in its effect on the autonomic nervous system. Telling your blood pressure to drop just doesn't do it. On the other hand, "the autonomic nervous system responds to a more basic language—imagery."[140]

Psychoanalyst Gerald Epstein believes that "People have to see that the mind, using imagery, can repair the body."[141] He reports the case of a man with chronic eczema who was given an exercise to do three times a day for three weeks. Detailed instructions included "imagining his fingers becoming palm leaves which he put on his face."[142] To finish the exercise he was to see his face becoming all clear. First the eczema moved from his face to his body and then cleared completely.

A woman with arthritis was given an imaging exercise that shrunk by 3 1/2 inches an eight-inch rheumatoid nodule in her right knee. A man facing prostate surgery had a normal prostate after doing a simple imagery twice daily for six months.[143]

Using mental imagery may even enhance visual perception. According to research psychologist Ronald Finke, you might see something more quickly if you first imagine it. "Suppose you are flying an airplane through a cloud, you might see the runway sooner if you were to imagine it in advance at its proper location. If on the other hand, you imagined it at a different location, you might take longer to see it correctly than if you had not imagined it at all."[144] You see what you believe and if you don't believe it, you may not see it.

Polar Bears Can Chill Cancer

Erik Esselstyn is a living example of the effectiveness of visualization and facing emotions in the long-term cure of cancer. He has been cancer free for more than 20 years. He tells the following story:

"In 1976, I developed bile duct cancer, a rare form of cancer, difficult to diagnose and treat. Extensive surgery removed the cancer and parts of my stomach, pancreas, duodenum, gall bladder and common bile duct.

"The prognosis after this surgery was poor so, after reading about visualization as a weapon against cancer in the Simontons' book *Getting Well Again*, I began to do visualization twice a day for twenty minutes. First I would use a mantra-based meditation to relax and to release static energy from my system. Then I would visualize an army of white polar bears I recruited to assist me in my cancer battle. I saw countless imaginary polar bears coursing through my bloodstream and lymphatic system, always on the lookout for cancer cells, always ready to devour them.

"I chose the polar bears because they are brave, resolute hunters, and persistent survivors. Their white color clearly relates to the body's white blood cells. Trooping through my system they searched out and devoured any lingering cancer cells. Other images could work, but the white polar bear, warm and fuzzy in my mind, remains a lifelong friend and ally searching out the dark, 'grapefruit-sized' cancer cells.

"For two years after the surgery I would feel/sense the polar bears zapping the ugly cancer cells. I knew each time another cancer cell was gone. At the end of each visualization session, the victorious polar bears met at the top of my brain, with thumbs-up for victory.

"I have continued this procedure since leaving the hospital in 1976. After two years I stopped feeling the sensation I called, 'a cancer cell being zapped.' My polar bears no longer encounter any of the grapefruit-sized menaces. While I believe all traces of the disease are gone, I still continue the visualization twice daily, sending my polar bear army on its mission through my system as a precaution against disease. The malignancy has never recurred. I am deeply grateful to the surgeon who performed the lifesaving surgery and to the Simontons for their self-help techniques."[145]

Another cancer patient visualized white knights on horseback running through her body, doing battle with the black cancer cells. The white knights symbolized antibodies at work. Another patient was a pacifist who refused to kill her cancer. She visualized herself carrying the malignant cells out of her body.

Besides eliminating errant cancer cells, visualization can help destroy bacteria and viruses, reduce tumors, heal broken bones and restore organic function in any part of your body. Visualization is also a preventive technique, stimulating immunity when used before overt signs of cancer or other disease. One can see the problem shrinking, burning up, erased, dissolved, or washed out of the body. Anecdotal reports, from a wide variety of sources, even credit visualization for helping individuals well-trained in the technique—in prevention or encouragement of conception.

Software for the Mind

Emmett Miller, M.D., founder and Medical Director of the Cancer Support and Education Center in Menlo Park, California, and author of the book *Self-Imagery*, specializes in psycho-physiological medicine and stress reduction. He created, *Source Cassettes* a series of audio cassette tapes—software for the mind—that provide the brain with clear, easy-to-comprehend "programs" designed to support self-healing, stress reduction, personal change, optimal performance and to prepare patients for surgery.

His deep relaxation/guided imagery audiocassette tapes are widely used by health professionals, business leaders, performers and athletes, including members of the U.S. Olympic Track and Field team. Many credit a significant portion of their healing and peak performance to these remarkable tapes, including folk music legend Joan Baez, and Olympic Decathalon Gold Medalist Dan O'Brien. Thousands more have learned to awaken their inner healer after receiving these enormously soothing and inspiring experiential cassettes from the Mayo Clinic, Kaiser Hospital, or their own personal health care practitioner. Years ago, I used the tapes regularly to prepare myself for surgery.

One patient used the surgery tapes before and after a radical hysterectomy and partial lymphectomy. She said, "The tape prepared me completely for what to expect, step-by-step; the shock and surprise were eliminated. The tape took me deep into my body and left me with a sense of well-being." Her surgeon called her recovery remarkable. Another used the surgery tapes before having a cancerous lung removed, a difficult operation for both surgeon and patient. Her doctor said that her recovery was the fastest he'd seen from this type of surgery.

Affirmations

Affirmations are consciously chosen seedthoughts one plants in the subconscious mind in order to produce a certain result. Dr. Miller explained:

"To change mental programming and create new, health-producing software, a key element is repetition. The unhealthy thought patterns were usually created over time, by your repeatedly thinking the same thoughts. To improve health, performance, and creativity you must think just as repeatedly in the newer way.

"Some of our requests to our brains are immediately followed by the appropriate behavior. Yet requests or demands to stop smoking, eat less, have a positive attitude, overcome a phobia of snakes, or stop feeling pain are seldom acted upon. This is because these behaviors—though felt consciously to be wrong—are stored unconsciously in the mind. When these same requests are offered as positive suggestions, images, and affirmations, they are more easily accepted, especially when the person has been guided into a relaxed, receptive state. In this state one is exquisitely receptive to new 'programs' which are offered in 'brain language'—positive affirmations, autosuggestions, and experience-based, sensory-rich imagery. We can improve our lives by making positive changes in our software."[146]

One man had his leg amputated below the knee. He had such great difficulty using an artificial leg that he couldn't walk. His skin kept ulcerating, causing a great deal of pain. During a hypnotherapy session he re-created the incident where his leg was lost, recalling his last thought as the leg was being blown off: "Now I'll never walk again." Using Miller's guided imagery tape he recreated the accident and imagined a different thought. He told himself repeatedly, "My leg is gone but I shall walk again using an artificial leg." He repeated this affirmation and saw himself walking. Within a few days of planting the new seedthought, the skin on his leg healed, he was freed from pain and he was able to wear the prosthesis.

Another patient used relaxation tapes to cure a hair-trigger temper. While in the relaxed state, he practiced dealing with difficult situations without anger. He rehearsed by first imagining provocative situations and then his calm reactions—many times over. At the end of each day, he reviewed every challenge to his calmness, praising his successes and visualizing a better way if he had handled the situation poorly. After a week, he reported major improvement in this behavior pattern.

Preparation for Surgery

There is a growing body of evidence that visualization and other mental techniques help prepare patients for surgery, and recover more quickly. "Researchers analyzed the results of over 190 studies of mental preparation for surgery and found that 80 per cent of the patients showed significant benefits: quicker recovery, fewer complications, less post-surgical pain, less need for pain medication, less anxiety and depression, and an average of 1.5 fewer days in the hospital."[147]

Victor W. Fazio, M.D., Chairman of the Department of Colon and Rectal Surgery at The Cleveland Clinic Foundation, found in his study of 130 surgery patients, those who used guided imagery left the hospital 1.5 days sooner, used half the pain medication, and returned to bowel functioning 1.2 days sooner than the control group. He also reported far less pre- and post-operative anxiety. He said, "We were surprised by the significant, measureable gains experienced by patients using guided imagery."[148]

Belleruth Naparstek, author of *Staying Well With Guided Imagery* is another pioneer in the field of guided imagery who has practiced pychotherapy for over 30 years. She is the creator of the Health Journeys series of over 20 disease-specific, guided-imagery-specific audio tapes, the tapes used in the Cleveland Clinic study mentioned above.[149] One of her success stories, Carol G., who began listening to the asthma tape after the potent combination of an asthma and a panic attack nearly killed her, has had great success in controlling her episodes. In fact she hasn't used her corticosteroids since.[150] I have successfully used her tapes and shared them with my meditation students. Be sure to include the use of audio cassette tapes in your Operating Manual tool kit.

Hypnosis

According to Hypnotherapist Linda Zelizer:

"Hypnosis is powerful, safe and easy to use. During hypnosis you are in an altered state, during which your critical conscious mind is less active and more open to changes. Hypnosis has helped many people to stop smoking, lose weight, overcome fears and phobias, reduce pain, eliminate insomnia, heal physical conditions, and improve both memory and concentration.

"Hypnosis works with your inner mind which influences everything you do. The power of hypnosis is in the mind's receptivity to suggestions during the altered state of awareness. You can then move past your learned limitations and focus your energy on new ways of thinking and behaving. You are never out of control so you won't say or do anything which goes against you. Hypnosis won't even make you do something you think you should do, but don't really want to do—like stop smoking..

"One technique, Hypnotic Exploration, used with a professional hypnotherapist, can help you to find the irrational thinking that is linked to the behavior you desire to change. Then in the hypnotically altered state, your chosen suggestions can help you to reprogram your beliefs and attitudes. Changing is then easier, more effective and more permanent. With such a potent resource, there's no longer a reason to believe that change is impossible."[151]

Pre-natal memories and birth trauma affect individuals well into adulthood, according to a growing body of research evidence. Hypnosis can help unlock the hidden memories so healing can take place. "Many people have recalled pre-natal and birth experiences that related to current physical and psychological problems: headaches, respiratory disorders, phobias, depression, anxiety. Recalling the experiences frequently relieves or eliminates the symptoms."[152]

A male client of therapist Jack Downing relived a painful fetal memory of rejection while under hypnosis. This was verified when his mother said that his father had indeed wanted her to have an abortion upon learning of the pregnancy.

Gynecologist David Cheek says his patients' ability to recall details of their birth is uncanny. He checks details, verifying their accuracy using obstetrical notes made during delivery. A researcher notes: "Patients' hypnotic recall of painful pressure to the head during birth is often enough to eliminate symptoms of chronic headache, including migraine. Cheek's patients commonly relate their reported birth experiences to present moods and behavior patterns. Many patients with asthma and emphysema were nearly suffocated during birth."[153] Understanding that *that was then, this is now*, helps these people change seedthoughts that are causing present-day distress.

Faith

Faith is accepting things unseen. It is believing without initial proof. Acting on a belief is evidence of faith! The proof or evidence people seek often comes after acts such as meditating, praying, chanting, visualizing or affirming. Anointing with oil, lighting a candle, and rain dancing are also actions people take to express their faith in something beyond themselves. These actions express one's faith in a Higher Power. Acting on faith may be the first prerequisite for healing yourself.

As a young mother when she was first diagnosed with Multiple Sclerosis, Psychotherapist Roberta Tager remembers crying out, "If there is a God, please hear me! I cannot have Multiple Sclerosis, these kids will need a mother! I cannot die when they are teenagers! My prayer was answered; my children are all grown and independent; I am free from MS symptoms; and that began my career in healing."[154] Roberta's faith at the time was limited but she still believed in the possibility that her prayer would be answered.

It's important to recognize that not everyone will be healed even with medical intervention. Certainly some people are healed without drugs or surgery. But for most others, medical interventions are an important part of their healing process. Not everyone is meant to be released from illness without medical treatment since illness is a growth and learning process which takes time.

A Zen monk once observed, "Healing begins in the mind." Faith in those words led my friend Martin to the attitude and behaviors that released him from cancer of the spinal cord. Even without the remission of his cancer, he became a happier person. Roberta Tager observes, "Now we have medicine, surgery, assorted body therapies, faith and love—perhaps the most important treatment there is. To quote my doctor husband, 'Spiritual healing can work hand in hand with medicine. It's another alternative.'"[155]

Regular weekly attendance at a church, synagogue or mosque can also serve as an expression of faith, as I have recently discovered. Previously I knew the power of personal prayer, and even the value of asking groups of others to pray for me. Still, for a long time I avoided participating in weekly religious worship services. Today, no matter how tough and stressful life gets, I now know that Shabbat, the Sabbath, the Biblical seventh day of rest and re-creation, arrives like clockwork. I then partake of the spiritual sustenance available to me during weekly worship services. When I made the commitment in 1992 and began to attend Services regularly, I experienced a sense of joy and contentment which really surprised me. Later I recognized a way of achieving an inner peace and healing which I may write about in a book with the working title of *The Worship Diary Process.*

Without some measure of faith most people wouldn't take the time to meditate, chant or do affirmations and visualizations. Faith plants life-affirming seedthoughts. If you are looking for ways to improve your life, *then you already have sufficient faith in a better future to do what it takes to create it.*

Sometimes people read statements like this and take them to mean that if they just follow the advice, they will be cured of whatever illness they have. That is not the way life works. No one can guarantee that the hoped-for result will occur. A cure may not always be the end result. In the case of Martin and Roberta, and others, a complete remission did occur. But at other times, the healing may consist of a release from negative emotions, or a feeling of inner peace.

In my case the tumor was removed, but damage remained in my body. Yet I still have a life that brings me satisfaction, fulfillment and happiness. Please avoid feelings of guilt, blame, self-doubt and rejection of helpful techniques if a complete cure isn't in the cards for you. Perhaps the best advice is *Expect the best and then take what you get and make the most of it.*

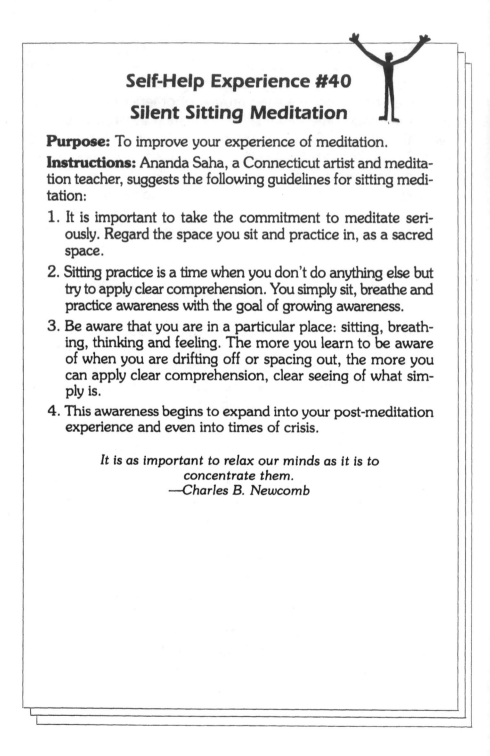

Self-Help Experience #40

Silent Sitting Meditation

Purpose: To improve your experience of meditation.

Instructions: Ananda Saha, a Connecticut artist and meditation teacher, suggests the following guidelines for sitting meditation:

1. It is important to take the commitment to meditate seriously. Regard the space you sit and practice in, as a sacred space.

2. Sitting practice is a time when you don't do anything else but try to apply clear comprehension. You simply sit, breathe and practice awareness with the goal of growing awareness.

3. Be aware that you are in a particular place: sitting, breathing, thinking and feeling. The more you learn to be aware of when you are drifting off or spacing out, the more you can apply clear comprehension, clear seeing of what simply is.

4. This awareness begins to expand into your post-meditation experience and even into times of crisis.

It is as important to relax our minds as it is to
concentrate them.
—Charles B. Newcomb

Self-Help Experience #41

Linda Zelizer's Guidelines for Self-Hypnosis and Creating Affirmations

Purpose: General information to help you create effective affirmations—to create the conditions you want to appear in your life. This simple but powerful technique makes change easier, by tapping into both the intuitive and rational sides of your brain.

The subconscious mind can be a garden where you plant seeds, or a weed field left to chance. An affirmation is a powerful pesticide, eradicating a harmful seedthought while allowing a desirable thought to grow and multiply. Outer conditions in your life reflect your inner reality, so willfully changing your inner reality produces good results. Focus your thoughts on specific intentions as an effective personal, or even political, change agent. Affirmations use words to guide you creatively toward the experience of well-being.

Affirmations can be *repeated aloud, thought silently* or even *written out daily* to reinforce the chosen programming you are offering your mental computer. Affirmations used with imagery are most effective. Some people draw pictures related to the intended result. *Affirmations are self-instructions.* Repeat them many times daily for several weeks in order to produce your desired result. Just as a magnet attracts metal, the thoughts you dwell in become the reality of your life. Right words, thoughts and action are needed for healing. Make these a part of your Operating Manual.

Instructions:

1. **Define something about yourself that you want to change.** Describe specific ways you would act when you reach your goal.

2. **Relax your body and your mind using any of the relaxation techniques described in this book.**

(continued) next page

3. After you reach the relaxed state, use visualization to imagine yourself reaching your goal. Mentally create that picture in great detail until you see or feel yourself feeling happy, having already made the change. *For example:*

- To lose weight, see yourself thin.
- To be able to speak comfortably in front of a group, imagine yourself speaking there.
- To eliminate a tumor from your body, first imagine it disappearing and then see your body without it.
- To improve your general level of health, imagine your body functioning in perfect health and harmony.

4. Design an affirmation which recognizes you at your goal. Use the present tense. *For example:*

- I feel healthy and alive.
- I concentrate effectively.
- My tennis game improves daily.
- I am stronger and healthier and more balanced each day.

Do not use the future tense, because it creates an inner mind program which says that you are not ready now. The present tense, affirms your readiness and willingness to reach your goal now. Keep the affirmation positive with the emphasis on you at your goal now.

One man read about hypnosis and began to affirm to himself, "I am *not* hungry." He actually gained weight. Each time he told himself "I am not hungry," he focused his attention inside to see if he was hungry. He thought about hunger so often that he put conscious energy into being hungry. He said that he was more hungry when he used an affirmation denying hunger than when he didn't think about hunger.

Telling yourself not to do something, you focus attention on the very thing you are avoiding, making it harder to avoid—try not to think about a pink elephant as you read this. For the affirmation to succeed, the mind and imagination must focus on the positive goal.

The wording you use is very important. You must use statements that your conscious mind can accept. *For example,* suppose you choose to work on your level of prosperity. To create wealth you decide to affirm, "I am a rich woman." This would be a wonderful affirmation if your conscious mind would believe the statement. If you are thousands of dollars in debt but affirm "I am a rich woman," your conscious mind might be thinking, "Oh yeah, who says you're rich, you're broke!" That would reinforce the negative state—a lack of prosperity.

In order for affirmations to work they must be reasonable, believable and acceptable to the conscious mind, lest the mind dismiss the affirmation as mere wishful thinking. The mind must hear an affirmation and really believe it could be true or become true.

5. **Stay with the positive image visualization and affirmation that you have created for several minutes.** In this relaxed state, allow yourself to feel good and enjoy the scenario. If you do not feel good with what you are doing, change your imaging until you do feel good. Strong feelings help to reinforce your beliefs. Strong negative feelings may keep you repeating the same negative behavior. Strong positive feelings will reinforce the positive behavior.

6. **To return to normal awareness, take a long deep breath and gently bring yourself back to consciousness of your present day environment.** Return to awareness with the good feelings you have created during your self-guided visualization.

I learned that nothing is impossible when we follow our inner guidance, even when its direction may threaten us by reversing our usual logic.
—Gerald Jampolsky

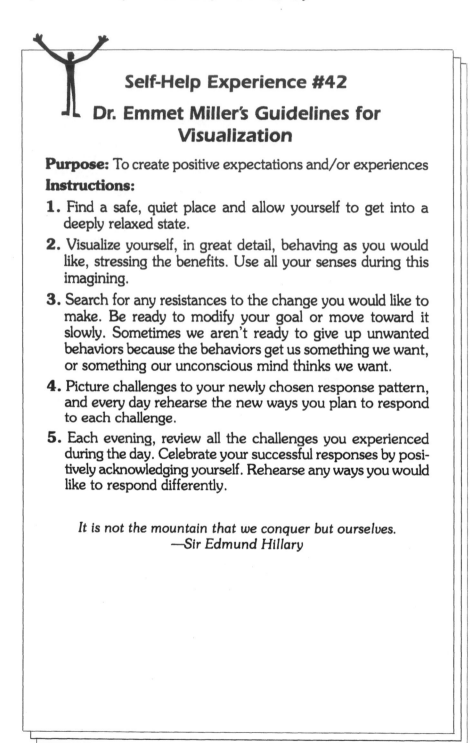

Self-Help Experience #42

Dr. Emmet Miller's Guidelines for Visualization

Purpose: To create positive expectations and/or experiences

Instructions:

1. Find a safe, quiet place and allow yourself to get into a deeply relaxed state.

2. Visualize yourself, in great detail, behaving as you would like, stressing the benefits. Use all your senses during this imagining.

3. Search for any resistances to the change you would like to make. Be ready to modify your goal or move toward it slowly. Sometimes we aren't ready to give up unwanted behaviors because the behaviors get us something we want, or something our unconscious mind thinks we want.

4. Picture challenges to your newly chosen response pattern, and every day rehearse the new ways you plan to respond to each challenge.

5. Each evening, review all the challenges you experienced during the day. Celebrate your successful responses by positively acknowledging yourself. Rehearse any ways you would like to respond differently.

It is not the mountain that we conquer but ourselves.
—Sir Edmund Hillary

Self-Help Experience #43

Biblical Scriptures As Affirmations and Change Agents

Purpose: To provide some scripturally-based affirmations.

Instructions: Some people are comforted reading the Bible— a dynamic self-help process. God's words are seedthoughts that grow into positive core beliefs when memorized and repeated regularly. Evangelist Kenneth Copeland says that "we take charge of our lives by taking complete charge of our tongues."

The following biblical verses are prescriptions for living, or promises from God.

- A soft answer turns away wrath, but harsh words cause quarrels. (Prov. 15:1)

- Reckless words pierce like a sword: but the tongue of the wise brings healing. (Prov. 12:18)

- A soothing tongue is a tree of life: but perverseness in it crushes the spirit. (Prov. 15:4)

- A cheerful heart does good like medicine, but a broken spirit makes one sick. (Prov. 17:22)

- God is our refuge and strength, a tested help in times of trouble. (Ps. 46:1)

- A relaxed attitude lengthens a man's life; jealousy rots it away. (Prov. 14:30)

- The wicked man's fears will all come true, and so will the good man's hopes. (Prov. 10:24)

- In those days when you pray, I will listen. (Jer. 29:12)

- I will give you back your health again and heal your wounds, saith the Lord. (Jer. 30:17)

- No, I will not break my covenant; I will not take back one word of what I said. (Ps. 89:34)

(continued) next page

- These are the blessings that will come upon you:

    Blessings in the city, Blessings in the field;

    Many children, Ample crops, Large flocks and herds;

    Blessings of fruit and bread;

    Blessings when you come in, Blessings when you go out. (Deut. 28:2-6)

- I have said I would do it and I will. (Is. 46:11)

- Therefore I tell you, whatever you ask for in prayer, believe that you have received it, and it will be yours. (Mark 11:24)

In my soul I know that God knows me and loves me,
and loves me even though he knows me. My heart has
every reason to smile.
—Greg Anderson

Good night, sweet prince.

Sweet dreams.

Chapter 14

Healing Through Dreamwork and Artwork

Through dreams you can communicate between your conscious and unconscious mind. This language connection uses symbols to take you to a space beyond your limited daytime awareness. The symbolism of the dream may initially escape your daytime mind's search for the meaning of your nighttime experience. Still, dreams are especially valuable because during sleep your conscious mind is turned down and its everyday judgments do not interfere. Then the dream can communicate what you need to know. You might get sick in an unconscious attempt to express your buried emotions. But through a dream you can rediscover and release stored emotional experiences in a helpful, healthful, benign fashion, making body illness unnecessary as a way of expressing emotions.

You can use sleep to heal yourself physically, emotionally, and spiritually. While dreaming you can work out fears, problems, negative emotions, and stressful relationships. These positive effects of sleep occur whether or not you remember dreaming.

Dreams provide you with an altered experience of reality, a different time and space reference. Scientific understanding of dream mechanisms is still in its infancy, though people have been turning to dreams for knowledge for centuries. Even the Bible speaks of prophecy divined through dreams.

The Metaphorical Language of Sleep

Here is an example of how I use my dreams. My "drilling dream" was short but very meaningful, and occurred on December 3, 1982.

"I dreamed Dr. Bernie Siegel was a dentist working on me. Drilling in my mouth, he worked from left to right. I don't remember the work on the left, but he drilled a lot on my right. He had me open my mouth wide."

I wrote the dream and the following interpretation in my journal:

"I thought a lot about this dream, wondering about the meaning. Is this a message about health, or death? Dr. Siegel deals with cancer and death. I've listened to his taped lectures and read his written material. Though I've never really worried about cancer, I do fear illness and think about dying. The right side of my mouth is a dream symbol for my unconscious emotions just as the right brain represents the intuitive and unconscious. Dr. Siegel symbolically digs out my emotions, digging them out of solid rock (the tooth). Am I resisting the idea of death? Right now I believe drilling (to get at my cavities) is a symbol of the effort I must expend to make permanent changes in my attitudes and emotions. I also realize that I am indeed making those changes—one step at a time—and have been for years. The process will accelerate because now I have a drill to follow and excellent helpers to practice with."

After making my initial notes, I continued to try to understand this dream, which touched me deeply. Later I added the following: "Since the right side represents the unconscious, a dentist drilling there could be drilling into my subconscious to retrieve the knowledge that is stored there (drilling to remove). Or the idea behind the symbol of a dentist drilling could be a metaphor related to practicing a drill, of me drilling till I am master of the material and have learned my lessons. The dream metaphor thus relates to education in the original Latin sense of 'drawing out,' and education in the modern sense of cramming in. Drilling is a word with two meanings in this context. On the one hand, Dr. Siegel was my teacher, drilling information into me. On the other hand, he was drilling to retrieve information— my healing knowledge and experiences that I want to share in my book."

This drilling dream was significant and I immediately knew it. The dream gave me direction via the seedthought (leave what's left and go right/write). I had the dream six months before I began the first draft of the first edition of this book. It confirmed what I would write (drill/retrieve/right) about. It also gave me the idea to ask Dr. Siegel and other professionals for help. Busy though he was, he gave me information, support, and encouragement.

Dreams can be prophetic. Two months after the drilling dream, I had dental work to remove an abscess on the root of a tooth on the right side of my mouth. This was the same spot where Dr. Siegel, as the dentist in my dream, was drilling. My bodymind, through the dream, prepared me for physical work I needed to help my body and save the tooth above the abscess. I was fortunate to have one of those rare dreams that transmits a message on many levels.

Dreams Reveal, Not Conceal

During a workshop, Dr. Montague Ullman, psychiatrist, co-author of *Working With Dreams* and founder of the Maimonides Hospital Dream Lab, provided some scientific background for my experience of dreams. He said:

"Dreaming is an activity we engage in regularly, during a profoundly altered state of being (as a natural part of the sleep cycle). The dream is a function of the sleeping state. When we waken we retrieve part of the experience of dreaming. The effort to recall the dream is an attempt to capture in ordinary language, an experience which has occurred in a different mode, a pictorial mode. The initial dreaming experience undergoes a transformation. During the process some information is lost.

"During dreaming we produce lots of imagery. The brain generates images every 90 minutes. That is, we begin to dream whether we remember the dream or not. This has been determined by years of laboratory research with many different subjects. Dreaming is a universal phenomenon which should and could be accessible to all. Dreams are important communications we aren't paying enough attention to.

"*The purpose of the dream is to reveal, not conceal.* We rearrange visual images to express feelings we are experiencing at the time. Expressed in this manner they have an emotional impact. Metaphors are comparisons between two different things that reveal an underlying identity more powerfully than through the ordinary use of language. Dreams are visual metaphors and sometimes metaphors are difficult to understand.

"Sometimes ideas about the meaning of a dream come after the lapse of some time. In many instances, on awakening, our dreams at first seem rather puzzling. Yet dreams shed light on our current life situation by helping us view the present from the perspective of the past. From that perspective, we may anticipate some things about the future, but we can't know the future. Dream work is healing in the sense of making us feel more whole."[156]

Dr. Ullman recommends working on understanding dreams with another person or group of people. I have sometimes found this helpful. The questions others ask on hearing about a dream, and the feedback the sharing generates, have been invaluable in my quest to know myself. The dream often re-arranges content from your current life within a new context. The altered perspective helps you view the present creatively. Don't talk about all your dreams, only those with such powerful imagery that they affect you emotionally. You will know the dreams whose meaning and metaphors need to be explored. Trust your intuition to lead you. Important dream messages will be repeated in different ways, until you get the message.

Interpret Dreams with Caution

Sometimes dreams foretell serious illness, or even death, for yourself or another. Dreams are then a helpful warning system. But because the dream is couched in symbolism and metaphor, the meaning can be unclear. Sometimes dreams of illness or even death symbolize other emotional processes that need exploration and healing. Don't take each such scary dream literally. Dreams must be viewed in the context of a total life situation for a clear meaning to emerge. Death dreams—subject to misinterpretation which increases fear—often don't relate to death at all but instead symbolize change.

Often death dreams have spiritual or emotional significance and indicate a change in the way the dreamer relates to the one who supposedly died. A teenager about to leave home or a woman wanting more independence from her husband might dream of a death in the family. Prior to leaving for college, my daughter Jennifer dreamed of my death on two occasions, which was at first frightening to us both. But the date she gave came and went quite a while ago, and I am still here. From a metaphysical point of view, dreaming of a parent's death is a way for adolescents to deal with the process of growing up and detaching from the parent. Dreams of your own death can signify rebirth into a new way of being. Perhaps a new, more appropriate behavior is about to be established with death to the old behaviors.

The beauty and difficulty of dreamwork is that messages come in symbolic form. If you think your dream means some trouble is brewing in your life, take heed. Perhaps the dream was meant to alert you to a problem which can be avoided by appropriate action, like the action Pharoah took in the Biblical story of Joseph, when he stored grain in anticipation of famine. Sometimes dreams reassure us like the dream of the biblical patriarch Jacob who recognized God's loving presence in his life after dreaming of angels going up and down a ladder.

Many books are available to assist you with the common, generic meanings of dream symbols. But I would encourage you to find your own meaning. After all, it's your dream, arising from your sleep consciousness, so you are best equipped to understand and interpret its meaning. By all means get feedback from others, but ultimately, *the buck stops with you.* It's up to you to decide on the meaning of the dream vis a vis your life.

J. Allan Hobson, a Harvard Medical School professor, is using students' dreams to acquaint them with the nature of another altered state—the psychotic experience. He said, "You can't hear it through a stethoscope and you can't see it on an X-ray. Furthermore, patients are reluctant even to give you a description of it. But we regularly experience in our dreams, mental states more similar to psychosis than anything a patient or I could describe in words." Hobson said that "every symptom of major mental illness is experienced in students' own dreams—disorientation, memory loss, bizarre thoughts, hallucinations, grandiosity, delusions and intense fear, rage, and euphoria."[157]

There is some evidence for a new kind of dream called a "breakthrough dream." According to psychologist Joseph Hart, clinical director at the Center Foundation in Los Angeles, "It's a lucid, powerful dream. The dreamer has full feeling and expression. There's vivid, total recall of the dream, and it invariably has a strong therapeutic impact on the dreamer. Lee Woldenberg, the center's medical director, described the dream as a bridge between the power, feeling, and creativity of the unconscious mind and the clarity and cognitive abilities of the conscious mind. We're impressed with the psychotherapeutic potential of this kind of dreaming and are developing ways to teach people to dream this way."[158] Besides help in healing oneself, dreams are reputed to have been involved in "breakthrough discoveries" in diverse fields of human endeavor, from scientific discoveries to ways of implementing new knowledge for the good of mankind.

Above all, relax. Enjoy your dreams. Often, they are as interesting as a good movie. Psychotherapist Dr. Stephen Aizenstat is an authority on dreamwork. He says, "Feces are one of the most engaging images. Feces are manure, manure means seeds, seeds mean growth. When feces appear in dreams.

I get hopeful. Right around the corner there's fertile ground for growth, new possibilities."[159]

Dr. Bernie Siegel—Teacher/Healer/ Dreamworker

Dr. Bernie Siegel, prolific, best selling author, lecturer and workshop leader is a former assistant clinical professor at Yale Medical School. Dr. Siegel, a surgeon now retired from private practice, has helped innumerable people with potentially fatal illnesses learn to live better and longer. These people, with cancer and many other life-threatening illnesses, participate in Exceptional Cancer Patient (ECAP) groups with other exceptional patients. Each one is willing to take an active part in, and responsibility for, his or her own healing. His writings describe a remarkable force: the healing power of love.

This smiling man, with the clean-shaven head, makes use of the dreams and drawings of his patients in the diagnosis and treatment of illness. His thesis is that spontaneous drawings, at critical moments in a person's life, are quite meaningful. As a surgeon, he could verify the diagnosis made on the basis of a patient's drawings. There appears to be a remarkable correlation between the intuitive diagnosis and the actual diagnosis, verified through medical/surgical techniques. It seems that the patient always knows, at some level of consciousness, what is going on in his or her body. The drawings are a way of moving past the conscious mind (which probably doesn't know), to the subconscious (which reflects its knowing in the drawings.) Dreams often serve the same function.

Dr. Siegel contends that patients, especially those with catastrophic illnesses, know the cause and course of their illness, at a deep unconscious level. They can retrieve this information through their dreams and drawings. If they are to alter the course favorably, change must occur at this deep level. Dr. Siegel recounts some fascinating experiences with dreams in the following article which he graciously agreed to have included in this book.

Dreams and Spontaneous Drawings[160]

By Bernie S. Siegel, M.D. and Barbara H. Siegel, B.S.

Physicians are generally trained as mechanics, with very little attention paid to the relationship between psyche and soma. Due to a personal search and growth process, as well as a congenial relationship with Elisabeth Kübler-Ross, I was exposed to the work of Susan Bach, an English psychotherapist and student of Carl Jung. Susan's work with spontaneous drawings led to my own.

As a practicing surgeon, I explored the active role of the mind in illness and was astonished at the information available via dreams and drawings. I became aware that patients knew their diagnoses. The mind literally knew what was going on in the body. When I shared my beliefs and was open, the patients began to share with me their knowledge of the future events and the outcome of their diseases and treatments. Now I routinely ask for dream material and for drawings as part of their care and as part of the diagnostic testing process.

Dreams

A patient with breast cancer reported a dream in which her head was shaved and the word "cancer" written on it. She awakened with the knowledge that she had brain metastases. No physical signs or symptoms appeared until three weeks had passed, when the dream diagnosis was confirmed.

Another patient had a dream in which a shellfish opened and a worm presented itself. An old woman points and says, "That's what's wrong with you." The patient, a nurse, sick with an undiagnosed illness, awakens with the knowledge that hepatitis is her diagnosis. Her physician confirmed the diagnosis.

I Turn to Drawings

In view of my own limitations as a dream analyst, I have turned to drawings, which like the unconscious material in dreams, can be interpreted for diagnosis and appropriate therapy.

Guidelines created by Susan Bach, assist in the drawing interpretation. Drawings have accurately predicted the time, and cause, of death. Remember I am dealing with many severely, sometimes terminally, ill patients.

I ask patients to draw or symbolize themselves, their disease, their treatment, and their white blood cells. Then a new realm of information is presented to us. The dreams and drawings reveal the vital nature of our life processes. It is not only our emotions which come to the surface symbolically, but also our somatic and intuitive processes.

In drawing one's self, or using symbols of the self, such as birds, trees, or houses, we portray our unconscious knowledge of present and future. A quite sick four-year-old draws a purple balloon floating up into the sky, with her name on it. There are multicolored decorations around the balloon, plus a shape which resembles a cake. This child died on her mother's birthday.

A young man with a brain tumor (whose recent tests were all negative) drew a tree that looked exactly like the profile of a brain. The tree showed black throughout, suggesting to me recurrent cancer, which was subsequently detected by CAT scan.

Predicting the Results of Treatment

The future results of chemotherapy and surgery can also be revealed in drawings. If patients see their treatment as an insult, assault, or poison, they react accordingly, often suffering side effects. On the other hand, the unconscious mind which believes in and accepts the therapy, alters the side effects and produces a better therapeutic result. This information is important so that we may alter any negative beliefs before treatment.

One patient drew X-ray therapy as black and red arrows spraying his body. He had a terrible reaction to the therapy. The drawing represented a negative expectation and the patient's belief was fulfilled.

Another patient drew X-ray therapy as a golden beam of energy. This patient had an excellent result with no side effects. The drawing represented a positive self-fulfilling prophecy. This patient had peace of mind which presaged healing. "Scientific" changes occur in the body when we have peace of mind.

Improving the Effects of Treatment

One of the most significant examples was a man who left his doctor's office when he was told the treatment would kill his cancer. He was a Quaker, a conscientious objector, and never killed anything. His drawing had been of little men carrying away his cancer cells. He is alive several years later, using his mind and vitamin C as healing agents.

An important point to be aware of is the difficulty our mind/body encounters as medicine wages a war on disease. The language of treatment is often depressing to the patient. Our bodies are the battleground, and the fact is that only a small percentage of people (15–20%) are comfortable being aggressive (killing the disease). The others manifest unconscious rejection of the treatment because of its association with destruction and killing. Physicians need to present the treatment as an aid to the healing process rather than as death to cancer or a war on disease.

Elisabeth Kübler-Ross emphasized the importance to me of "Thou shalt not kill" as a commandment in our conscious and unconscious minds. I have received drawings from patients with the cancer saying, "Help!" On other drawings the white blood cells look like popcorn so that they won't hurt the disease. *The mind is aware that the disease is us.*

I learned that we need to love ourselves in order to heal. The love stimulates our immune system, and white blood cells, to work for us. The effects of love and despair have been verified in studies of immune responses to various stimuli. We must learn to consume the disease by using it as nourishment... ingesting the disease as our white blood cells do, using it as a source of psychological growth. We learn ways to improve ourselves and love fully from disease. Disease leads to correcting an imbalanced pattern in the system. For some, disease can be seen as a healing of the soul.

Medical mechanics do not often realize the importance of patients' belief systems in the outcome of therapy. If we are to achieve exceptional results we must start working to unite the team of mind, body, and spirit. The dream process and visualization help us do this.

Dreams Guide Treatment

A patient listening to his inner voice often receives instructions via dreams or during meditation. One man who recovered, was asked to take injections of vitamin C and to utilize computer images for positive subliminal stimulation. Exploration of these techniques has just begun by orthodox medicine. It seems the inner voice preceded the medical profession in exploring the path to self-healing, or participation with the physician.

A woman was in severe pain and was told by a voice (she called it the Holy Spirit) that she had appendicitis and had better go to the Emergency Room. She said that she wanted to wait, but the voice insisted she go. My diagnosis simply confirmed her pre-existing knowledge.

As I have explored the nature of healing and have moved further from the mechanistic medical model, principles have arisen tying together many so-called mystical events. The body is not a machine but is a vibrant system of physical and electrical energy whose tissues and organs have their own frequencies and cycles, their own rhythms. The nervous system becomes the transmitter of this information to the conscious mind.

When a salamander loses a limb or a tail it is aware of the loss and it communicates with the injured part. It "listens" to the nerves in that area and answers by initiating regeneration.

Disease states represent an alteration in the pattern within the human energy system. If one "listens," the symptoms present themselves. For some, these symptoms, or this awareness, is through physical signs. But for many, the message comes via dreams, intuition, and the unconscious or spontaneous drawings which can be interpreted.

When I began to utilize the picture drawing technique in my surgical practice, I was able to see within the drawings the intimate relationship between psyche and soma. Also revealed to me was invaluable information stemming from the unconscious and from the individual's intuitive awareness.

In summary, may I say that this exposure has led me to believe that the psyche and soma are communicating and that somatic problems can be brought to consciousness via symbols. Also, I believe as Carl Jung did, that "the future is unconsciously prepared long in advance and therefore can be guessed by clairvoyants."

These experiences have shown me a new path as a healer, teacher, care giver, and have reinforced my beliefs. My patients now feel free to share experiences they would never share with a mechanistic M.D.—one who sees only the mechanical process of disease in the body, without recognizing the totally integrated role of the mind and emotions.

Self-Help Experience #44

To Sleep, To Dream, To Remember

Purpose: To help in remembering your dreams.

Instructions:

1. You can improve your ability to remember dreams. Suggest to yourself at bedtime that you will recall a dream upon arising. "I will remember a dream." Remembering is a choice you make. Forgetting is also a choice, a choice that perhaps you have forgotten you made.

2. If you have a specific situation you are working on, before going to sleep ask God, a Higher Power, or your Inner Wisdom for guidance related to that problem.

3. Keep a pencil and paper by your bedside to make note of any thoughts or images upon awakening. Allow time to wake slowly in the morning. If you recall a dream, tell yourself about it, to anchor it in your memory. Then write it down.

4. If no dream images or memories arise, notice what you are thinking about. Write down your thoughts. They might not be of a dream, but your nighttime experiences will have led to your awakening thoughts which may or may not be useful to you. Take your dream journal with you if you leave home in the morning. Sometimes a dream is remembered later on.

5. If you still have trouble remembering a dream, think back to the last dream you remember having and try to analyze that. Often discovering an old dream's hidden meaning will enable you to move on to a new area in your life, with a new sequence of dreams.

6. Remember, you are the maker of the meaning in your life. A dream symbol may be meaningful to you alone. It's up to you to find if there are any significant connections between your thoughts, your daily life, and a specific dream.

It is better to be prepared for an opportunity and not have one than to have an opportunity and not be prepared.
—Whitney Young, Jr.

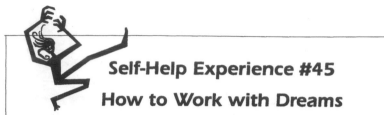

Self-Help Experience #45

How to Work with Dreams

Purpose: To improve the benefits you receive from your dreams.

Explore the meaning of a dream through questions you ask yourself. Questions help you to discover what present life context shaped the dream. If you know how the dream relates to your present life you may learn about changes in your life that are necessary. The relationship of a dream to your present life isn't always easily accessible. But those vivid dreams that are filled with shocking or stimulating imagery generally have meaning that you can discover and use.

Sometimes it's helpful to share the dream with another person to get another impression. Often the reactions of the listener shed light on the meaning of a dream. At times, I've found that the symbols in my dream mean more to my listener than to me.

Once I dreamed of bodies piled on railroad cars. The reaction of the therapist I shared it with was much stronger than my own. Another time I dreamed about a man I'd worked with having his legs blown off during a war. That dream was for both of us. The message: "Being forced to your knees is a symbol of humility." I think that sometimes we might actually be dreaming for other people's benefit.

There are books written about the universal meaning of various dream images and symbols. The information may help. Trust your intuitive voice to tell you what your symbol means to you. You'll know when you've made the right interpretation by the reaction of your body. Perhaps you'll feel a tingle or some other physical sensation announcing a perfect fit.

Instructions

1. Trust yourself! Make a commitment to work with your dreams, and your internal wisdom will guide you into understanding the message.

2. Write down your dream.

3. Give your dream a title.

4. Notice any striking images and ask yourself what they might mean. Pay special attention to recurring images, be they people, animals, places, colors or things.

5. Ask yourself, "What current event in my life is connected to this dream?"

6. Ask yourself, "What is this dream trying to tell me?"

7. Wait several hours or even a few days and then re-read what you wrote about your dream. Sometimes you will have forgotten the original dream. Then your written words are often more meaningful. Sometimes, my dream means nothing to me until I read what I wrote and then it almost seems like a direct message for me to do something. For example, I might write down, "I was traveling on the right road." Those kinds of notes confirm what I am doing in life.

8. As you re-read your dream notes, pay attention to any thoughts you are having. Inspirational messages often come while re-reading dream notes.

9. If you want to work in depth with dreams, read a book and/or join a group devoted to dreamwork.

> *Throw your dreams into space like a kite, and you do*
> *not know what it will bring back—a new life, a new*
> *friend, a new love, a new country.*
> *—Anaïs Nin*

Work hard, hang tough, and go the distance.

Think for yourself.

Honesty is the best policy.

Once burned, twice shy.

God be with you.

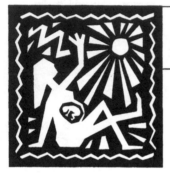

Chapter 15

Creating a New Context: Healing from Within

In chronic or recurrent acute illnesses your lifestyle is often key to your state of health. Lifestyle includes how you "language" your life: your attitude, thoughts, emotions, and style of thinking. You can create conditions more favorable to health by removing unhealthy negative belief systems. To be permanently effective, healing must occur in the mind.

The body acts out thoughts and images. Usually you aren't aware of this process in much the same way that you aren't usually conscious of breathing and other automatic body functions. But just as you can bring consciousness to bear on the process of breathing (choosing to breathe deeply, for example), you can positively influence many aspects of your body when you choose to pay attention.

Why Am I Sick? Because...

When thoughts and images are consciously chosen, the mind can create a context for health. A context is a frame of reference, a milieu, or an environment within which you operate. To recognize your present context, pay attention to those "why" questions you ask yourself, and listen to the different "becauses" you answer. Notice too your "why nots," "buts," and "if onlys." These connect to beliefs about the way things *should be* for us to be happy. The "becauses" are beliefs about what makes people sick. These beliefs can be harmful. Your health context contains all the beliefs that keep those "becauses" in place. Many of the contextual beliefs that can harm you are buried in your unconscious. Asking "why" can bring them out and lead you to more aware behavior.

Do you believe something will happen to you if you sleep less than eight hours, if you don't use rain gear, if you eat so-called junk food? Then perhaps you do need to get enough sleep, wear a raincoat and boots and eat better. Does the missed sleep or the lack of raingear or the junk food make you sick or do your beliefs about them cause you to be sick? Not everyone gets sick when they don't get enough sleep or when they get their feet wet or when they eat so-called unhealthy foods. Most people believe what they see. But, you will often see it because you already believe it. *Healing from within requires you to discover what you already believe and how those beliefs affect you.*

You can reduce the power of harmful beliefs and create a more favorable health context by using affirmations as seedthoughts planted in your body/mind. For example, "I am generating health because I say so" puts healing forces in motion. I created a favorable context for my own healing by continually affirming this seedthought among others consciously chosen , "I am grateful to my pure and perfect body for all it teaches me."

Shelly Bruce, one of the early stars of the original musical "Annie," was happy and successful. Then, suddenly she was diagnosed as having leukemia. In her book, *Tomorrow Is Today*, she describes her illness and provides an example of altering context. During her difficult hospitalization she was playing the part of victim to the hilt, while slowly being destroyed by forces she felt were beyond her control. Eventually, she realized that as a performer there was another way to play her life/role. She could play it like Annie, be master of her fate, and emerge triumphant.

Shelly Bruce created a new context when she said she was no longer a victim and chose to be an optimist. She rejected her fear and embraced a more positive future, one filled with hope. Her faith was quickly rewarded when she received her first visible sign of improvement—no leukemia cells after her next bone marrow test.

She created a more positive *context* in which to hold the *content* of her life, which was her case of leukemia. The last I heard, Shelly Bruce remained free of leukemia and was again performing. A miraculous beneficial side effect of her transforming self-improvement work was improvement in her singing voice. The transformation she experienced is available to you. "Miracles" are natural occurrences to those with faith and health-producing belief systems.

Since we do learn from adversity, that which seems to block us from our fervent desires may actually be there for our highest good. Sometimes we have lessons to be learned and knowledge of the self to gain before we can be healed. I now clearly see the benefits from my own prolonged healing before and after brain surgery. Learning patience and faith was a blessing. Learning to release envy and self-pity were gifts to myself, among many others—all growth resulting from my tumor. It often takes the passage of time to recognize the gifts or benefits to be gleaned from a difficult experience. But recognition of those benefits turns the difficult situation into a blessing that generates a new healing context within.

After I was released from the hospital, while still unable to drive, I saw my friend Pat. She had had a mastectomy several weeks earlier and had to be concerned about the cancer recurring. Unlike Pat I had no concern that my benign tumor would metastasize, so in that sense I was lucky. But she was up and around and really seemed fine, while I was still struggling, walking with a cane, barely able to focus my eyes, unable to talk above a whisper. I envied Pat and felt very sorry for myself.

Several months later Pat's cancer recurred. She developed brain cancer and suffered many of the symptoms I had. I quickly realized the futility of envy. Pat died a difficult death from cancer a year after that "pity party" I held for myself. And a dozen years later, I am still alive and doing well. Pat taught me a profound truth: Don't envy anyone. You never know what they will have to bear. Just be grateful for what you have.

Tumors and Diabetes

Dorothy Thau is a holistic health counselor who supports her patients in healing from within, teaching them to alter unhealthy contexts by recognizing and changing seedthoughts and core beliefs. She recounts this story:

"I had a 42-year-old patient with non-malignant intrauterine tumors. After fourteen months they were the size of a four-month pregnancy. This patient wanted to know why she had the tumors.

"In the first session I taught her visualization using guided imagery. During the session she was surprised to see the growths not as tumors but as an embryo, as if she was creating another child. She realized that subconsciously she felt that she had never completed her duty as a female. She would have liked to have had more children. The connection between her desire and the uterine problem surprised her. At last she understood her emotional connection to the tumors. She needed to forgive herself and release her guilt feelings related to 'no more children.'

"During her second session, I gave her these affirmations to use during her daily visualizations: 'My love and commitment to children can be fulfilled through my teaching career, as well as through my own two children. The job of my uterus is complete and it can relax and stop trying to create anything new.' She left with tools to alter her negative beliefs, feeling relieved and more relaxed."[161]

Dorothy Thau also described her work with another patient, a 56-year-old woman with diabetes who used insulin daily:

"Her goal was to halt the progression of her illness. During our work her circulation and eyesight improved and her use of insulin was drastically reduced.

"A breakthrough occurred after a treatment session where we used the technique of Age Regression Therapy. I regressed her eleven years to the onset of her disease, coinciding with her divorce from her husband. She recalled, 'I felt the sweetness had gone out of my life.' She then saw the connection between her illness, diabetes, and her emotions surrounding the divorce.

"She made rapid progress as she worked at letting go of any negative feelings about her ex-husband and the divorce. She affirmed, 'I feel positive about myself and my talents. I can live a sweet and fruitful life, in perfect health.'

"After completing the treatment, her personality changed. She is now in terrific shape. A prolific artist and art teacher, she puts in long hours and smiles continually. The sweetness has returned to her life! Previously, she had thought of herself as a 'diabetic,' living with that label, seeing herself as diseased and disabled. She no longer considers herself limited or diseased, certainly a dramatic *reversal of the context* in which she previously saw herself."[162]

According to Connecticut endocrinologist Dr. Bob Lang, "People with diabetes often express the perception that 'there is no sweetness in life.' That thought is often stress-inducing. Recurrent negative thoughts may be responsible for triggering illness or worsening an existing disease condition."[163]

Researchers at the University of Pittsburgh are studying the effects of shocks on the immune system. They report that there is often an association between the onset of diabetes (the content) and a separation, divorce, or the death of a parent (the context).[164]

Backbone

Hypnotherapist Linda Zelizer treated a woman with severe back problems who chose to explore the related emotional components. Zelizer's client remembered the words her mother used frequently before her death: "When I die, I want you to be the backbone of this family." She was already feeling pressured in her life. She did not want to be "the backbone" of her family. She realized that while she had always had some back problems, their severity increased dramatically when her mother died.

She found it easier to use her physical problems to avoid unwanted tasks than to say "No" and deal with the consequences. The payoff for her ill-health was avoidance of responsibilities.

Understanding the relationship of her physical distress to the seedthought "be the backbone of the family" led her to change her behavior, thus easing her backache problems.

But Zelizer says, "I've seen many cases where a payoff or secondary gain is an obstacle to the patient's getting well, and might be the reason for the unwanted behavior in the first place. Patients usually aren't aware of this payoff. Sometimes people come for hypnosis to change a specific habit and a deeper, underlying issue surfaces. Although they want to change the habit at one level, they are not always willing to deal with the deeper level. Sometimes they have some emotional investment in not solving the problem. Hypnosis is a wonderful tool but it is not magic."[165]

Another Zelizer patient was a young boy with recurrent ear infections and difficulty in hearing. He told Zelizer that he often said to himself, "I don't want to listen to you" when thinking about his verbally abusive father. They explored ways he could handle his father's put-downs. The boy learned to assert himself by telling his father "I don't like what you say." He used his imagination to create his relationship with his father getting better. He realized that his father's treatment of him related to the father's own bad feelings about himself. The new payoff was far fewer ear infections and improved hearing.

The Authentic You

Dr. Bernie Siegel's approach to healing is partly based on the concept that people's illnesses result from living lives that are not in accord with their authentic selves. Then conflict, stress, and negative emotions that disrupt the body's ability to control disease are generated. Fortunately, when people begin to act authentically, they can often reverse the process. Dr. Siegel helps people—with so-called fatal illnesses as well as "serious/chronic" ones—learn to live better and longer. Life-threatening becomes life-enhancing as he teaches patients how to achieve peace of mind and better health by understanding and loving themselves. In treating patients, Dr. Siegel used the orthodox medical tools, from surgery to chemotherapy, to remove cancer. But he knows that a dose of loving attention, from oneself and others, is a powerful healing force.

To create a health-ful context and effect inner healing, it is helpful to know what the patient unconsciously believes about his illness and its recommended treatment. Bernie's patients' drawings were a vital element in the healing process. Often the material gleaned from drawings leads to an alteration of the disease context. If the drawings reveal their perception of the treatment to be an attack, they often suffer side effects. So he first worked with his patients on reversing negative information stored in the unconscious.

This change of context, from focusing on the outer manifestations of disease to looking at the inner perceptions, has totally changed Siegel's life. It gave him a renewed sense of fulfillment in his profession, as well as vastly increasing his impact on those he serves. Even though he is retired from private practice his influence on the general public continues to grow through his best-selling books, TV appearances, lectures and workshops. By discovering his own authentic self, Dr. Bernie Siegel has pointed thousands of others towards discovering the authenticity of themselves.

Creating a Health-Full Context

Many years ago, President John F. Kennedy created a context for the success of the United States space program by *saying* that the United States was committed to a man walking on the moon in ten years. Kennedy gave his word when he created that commitment for all of us—to put a man on the moon. To regain and maintain good health requires commitment too. Take a stand! Give your word! Promise to work towards good health! Giving your word is evidence of your commitment to your goal, a big part of the language connection. You make the agreement, a promise to fulfill, a resolution you will keep. Love and accept yourself. Be alert to the process without attachment to the end result. If you learn from your experience, you are always a success, never a failure.

I have a context for my life that is large enough to include many aspects—self-confidence, worry, negativity, a positive outlook, joy, sorrow, pain, limitations, illness, and health. I attempt to make the most of each day. Sometimes I worry about various bodily sensations, but I always believe that essentially I am okay. Helpful images are those that represent life the way we want it to be. Images of suffering may be useful warnings, but aren't valuable as places to dwell. Since we attract to us that which we dwell on, I pay attention to warnings of doom, but dwell on positive, uplifting, health-producing images. When I relax and stop worrying about my bodily sensations, I feel and see myself healthier, and often become my good health.

Psychotherapist Roberta Tager sums up what I believe inner healing is all about. She says:

"I believe that the sole reason for bodily discomfort is so that our soul may learn. My body is the vehicle for my soul. Learning can take place at a very rapid rate. When one walks through life with an eye for the whole, one can step gently and correct each wrong step quickly. We each have chosen our lessons, only we have forgotten that we chose them.

"The enslavement of my soul has ended, and the learning and growth I chose is now available to me. Understanding attitudinal lessons is my way to release illness. The answer always lies within easy reach through meditation. Wellness is the natural state of the body. Releasing faulty thoughts allows wellness to return. This in no way negates the helpfulness of medical, surgical, or nutritional assistance."[166]

Forgiveness: How Do I Forgive?

Healing from within often requires a willingness to forgive oneself and others. Jacqui Bishop and Mary Grunte's gem of a book *How To Forgive When You Don't Know How* sheds light on what forgiveness is, clears up what it is not, evokes the desire to forgive and shows it's possible no matter what. They teach that forgiveness really helps the forgiver, not just the forgiven. Forgiveness plays a crucial role in freeing up our lives from suffering. Altering the context through which one views an experience facilitates inner healing.

Bishop and Grunte write, "...many people have concluded that all experience can provide soil for producing good fruit."[167] Often, the best way to forgive a wrong done is to learn something of value from the experience. One woman wrote how she forgave the man whose dishonest practices resulted in the loss of her husband's business. She soon recognized that her buried emotion about the bankruptcy and her anger that her husband's new job kept him away from home all week was "a prescription for disease and could lead to a major unwanted illness."[168] Then her transformation began. She wrote:

> "One day, I began to see that the situation was actually producing some gains in my life. For example, I no longer feared living alone. In fact, I was enjoying the freedom to do what I wanted, when I wanted. I could say I hated my new life or I could be really grateful for the lessons I learned and for the release from my former fear. I could choose to be happy—no matter what. Recognizing what I gained made it easier to forgive the man who stole from my husband. I am grateful to have found the key to turning life's lemon experiences into sweet, thirst-quenching lemonade."[169]

As this woman learned, true healing means knowing that ultimately we all die, and that during our life we will each face trials and tribulations. True healing is living within your circumstances and learning every step of the way. True healing means sometimes having to forgive others as well as yourself. True healing is going through the process awake, aware, alert, with acceptance, love, and joy. True healing means living your life as both actor and audience: you as the performer and you as the objective observer each can enjoy the show. True healing is concerned with the experience, not attached to the end result. If it works and an illness is reversed or a life saved, great! If not, at least you know you "made the most of it."

Self-Help Experience #46
Writing Yourself to Wholeness

Purpose: To keep track of experiences, uncover emotions, materialize what you want, and avoid what you don't want.

Instructions:

1. Write your feelings in your journal. Notice what makes you happy and what makes you feel upset. Write down any discoveries you make about yourself. For example, I found out I feel happier all day if I get up early and start working, even though I prefer to sleep late in the morning. Or, I need less sleep if I stay up late and sleep more soundly.

2. "Awfulize" and catastrophize any problem by imagining and writing down the worst that can happen. Read it aloud. See your worst case as absurd. Cross it out. Laugh it away.

3. Record your dreams.

4. List goals for a week, a month, three months, one year, five years, and ten years. Goals can be specific to fitness and health. For example:

   • I will lose 25 pounds this year.

   • I will improve my cardiovascular system by decreasing my resting pulse 10 beats.

   Include goals that support your psychological health as well. These could relate to work, relationships, and money, among others.

5. Choose a specific health-related area to work on. Write an affirmation regarding that area.

6. Write about any experience that you want to let go of, perhaps something that made you very sad or angry. After writing it down you can store it away. Then you can stop thinking about it but still have the details filed away. Or, you can tear it up and flush it down the toilet; or even burn the paper. Each of these writing-it-down rituals has worked for some people.

If the heart is bitter, sugar in the mouth won't help.
—Jewish Proverb

Self-Help Experience #47

Visualization for Strengthening the Immune System

Purpose: To rid your body of unwanted organisms.

The immune system contains white blood cells patrolling the body through the blood and lymphatic systems. There are two main types: T cells, produced in the thymus gland, are killer cells which destroy invading bacteria and viruses; B cells, produced in the bone marrow, neutralize poisons made by disease organisms while helping the body mobilize its own defenses. The immune system is controlled by the brain, either directly through the nerves and neurochemicals or indirectly through hormones in the bloodstream. Immunological changes can take days or weeks, unlike many other autonomic or hormonal changes that can take seconds or minutes.

According to one theory, cancer cells often appear in the body and are destroyed by white blood cells before they grow into dangerous tumors. When the immune system becomes suppressed and can no longer deal with this routine threat, cancer or some other disease might develop. So too, if the brain's control of the immune system is compromised, ill health might follow. Conversely, whatever strengthens your brain's control of your immune system will probably improve your health.

In this exercise, you send symbolic warriors-helper symbols to stimulate your immune system and aid your white blood cells in ridding your body of any intruding organisms. Use this for any infection, allergy, growth, or tumor. Some immune-enhancing agents might be white knights, doctors in white coats, Pacmen, polar bears, warfare weapons, vehicles like tanks or garbage trucks, squirt guns, lasers or phasers, and the letters T and B. You might prefer to use weapons of love, like valentines or a laser beam of golden light as your immune strengthening healing symbols. Be creative and think for yourself.

Instructions:

1. Relax into the helpful alpha state—awake though relaxed.

2. Choose your helper symbols and imagine them traveling throughout your entire body. Imagine them removing any unwanted organism.

3. When you are finished, thank your helpers for the work they did. Tell yourself, "This process strengthened my immune system."

4. Practice this with eyes closed, seated or lying down. When you get good at this you most likely will be able to do it with your eyes open.

There is no journey to healing. Healing is the journey.
—Greg Anderson

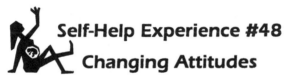 **Self-Help Experience #48**
Changing Attitudes

Purpose: To leave an unwanted situation or relationship without self-righteousness; to uncover your beliefs and change your attitude.

Instructions:

1. Write a sentence describing the unwanted situation or relationship and then list the reasons for disliking it. Underline those words or phrases that seem to have a strong emotional charge. Ask yourself the following questions related to the unwanted situation or relationship:

   • What is my core issue that is being challenged?

   • What reasons do I give myself to support my angry and hostile attitude?

   • Is my current attitude justified?

(continued) next page

- Do I want to change my attitude?
- Must I maintain my current attitude in order to leave this relationship or can I leave without rancor because it no longer serves my highest good?

People often make another person or thing wrong, in order to justify their current point of view. This self-righteous thinking often leads to hostile words and harmful behavior. For example, people often bad-mouth a relationship that they want to leave. They attack the other person in their thoughts and words. This leads to continuing hostility and angry feelings.

There is no need for you to attack that which isn't right for you in order to leave. You don't have to justify what you do by harming someone else even in your thoughts. There may be some situations where it is necessary to present your point of view about another, but in general this isn't necessary. More helpful languaging is to think and/or say, "This situation/relationship is not appropriate for me right now. I choose not to be here."

2. Pay attention to the reasons you give yourself for doing what you do. Evaluate the usefulness of thinking that way. Notice how your thoughts lead to your current attitudes. If you want to change your attitude, choose more appropriate thoughts.

3. Remember that another person's unjust criticism of you has power to harm you only if you allow it. *It's hard to fight an enemy who has an outpost in your own head.* No one can make you feel inferior without your own consent. Don't berate yourself for being who you are, thinking for yourself and feeling your feelings.

4. Repeating the words of this *prayer of St. Francis* has been helpful in transforming attitudes and creating a new way of seeing things:

> *Lord, make us instruments of Thy Peace.*
> *Where there is hatred, let us sow love,*
> *Where there is injury, pardon,*
> *Where there is doubt, faith,*

Where there is darkness light,
And where there is sadness, joy.
Grant that we may seek not so much to be consoled, as to
  console.
Not so much to be understood, as to understand.
Not so much to be loved, as to love.
For it is in giving that we receive.
It is in pardoning that we are pardoned.
And it is in dying that we are born to eternal life.

Self-Help Experience #49

The Daydreaming Exercise:
Imagining to Help the Planet

Purpose: To change your thinking and change your world.

We affect our health, as individuals, through the metaphors and beliefs evident in the stories that we tell ourselves. We can imagine sickness or we can imagine health.

In the same way, images and metaphors shared by members of a group, an organization, or a culture have a profound effect upon the group as a whole, as well as individuals within the group. We can imagine war, or we can imagine peace. You can imagine a worst case or a best case scenario. It's your choice.

Spend time imagining the whole world being the way you want it to be.

See it and believe it!

Instructions:

Close your eyes, visualize, pretend and make believe. You know how to do this!

Life is like a game of cards. The hand that is dealt you repre-
sents determinism; the way you play it is free will.
—Jawaharial Nehru

Make the best of it.

Practice what you preach.

Healer, heal thyself.

What you sow, you reap.

Keep on keeping on.

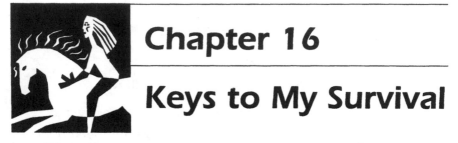

Chapter 16

Keys to My Survival

This chapter was written in response to a friend's questions: "What did you do to survive your brain surgery? What did you think, feel, and believe that helped you? What gives you strength that might inspire me?"

Writing the answers has been hard. But nonetheless, during that difficult process, I learned a lot about myself as I looked deep within and codified my beliefs. What I discovered was a real gift to myself. I notice that I'm more sure of myself and clearer about my core beliefs and opinions than ever before. Evidence continues to mount—from both my personal experience healing myself and my professional life researching and writing this book—for the existence of a mind/body link and the fact that language is a key connecting mechanism. I am clearer, too, about my personal language connections. When I am ill, I look for the connecting language and often discover my seedthought. The real inner me—the authentic me— is more accessible now.

36 Core Beliefs

I believe there is a Supreme Being, a God who guides and watches over me. I feel divinely protected. I have a personal relationship with that creative God force in the universe. That force is neither male nor female, but both, or all. I say "Mother/Father/God" when I pray. I believe God created each of us for companionship with each other and to receive God's blessings and love. A belief in a Supreme Being is often rejected by people until they reach a crisis and discover the power of prayer and faith. Faith activates healing.

I believe I am responsible for myself and say this often. I have a team of doctors who advise and treat me. As the captain of my team I make the final decision based on expert advice. I trusted Dr. Dogali, my neurosurgeon, and during surgery he was in charge. I believed he could help me and had faith in his treatment. During my post-surgical hospital stay, if I thought I needed something, I asked for it, sometimes quite forcefully. I fought for what I believed in. At least once, I was wrong. I admitted it.

I believe I am special and have a mission to accomplish. In 1985 I wrote a newsletter about my brain surgery. I shared it with hundreds of people. Sometimes I felt embarrassed when giving the letter to someone I barely knew. But if I thought I should share it, I did. The response from many people was favorable. I think they were inspired by me, as I was inspired by them. The personal stories these people told me often helped me to feel better about myself and encouraged me to "keep on keeping on."

I believe that I give meaning to the events in my life. I chose to survive in order to fulfill my purpose and complete my mission, part of which is to spread the information in this book.

I believe I can sometimes choose what to experience and sometimes I must take what I get. Some things are unavoidable, predestined, written in stone—my brain tumor probably was. But we do have some real choice.

I believe that we attract the experiences we need in order to learn. Since we have illness to learn something, I believe my growth and successful recovery from the tumor depended on choosing to learn from it.

I believe also that there is a randomness to the events in the universe. We can be in the right place at the right time, or the wrong place at the wrong time. I believe we are not to blame. Responsibility means accepting what happens without self-reproach, guilt, self-hate, or negativity.

I believe that we are not bad or wrong when we suffer pain or illness. Remember that!

I believe the main purpose of life is to learn. Life on Earth is like being in college. There are courses we take by attracting people and/or circumstances to learn from. We might not always like it. Perhaps we don't always choose the courses, but we do choose our receptivity to learning when the lesson appears. As part of the process, I use my body as a guide to uncover my emotions, thus learning from my body. Disease is sometimes a life-long learning process, rather than a distinctive one-time event.

I believe each illness teaches me something for my self-knowledge and is also part of my research for my books. During the early stages of my recovery I felt that I was proving myself and the message in this book. "Practice what you preach, Barbara, to learn what you teach" was a frequent seedthought of mine.

I believe illness or any crisis situation is a time of heightened potential. We may be more vulnerable, but then we have the chance to grow. As we say good-bye to the old ways, some part of us dies. You leave something you need to leave, in order to grow and move on. What we refer to as healing may just be us growing up. Perhaps a message of the great spiritual teachers from Moses to Buddha to Jesus to Mohammed is that there's no life without suffering and no joy without sorrow. The Bible teaches us that there is no promised land without an exodus, no resurrection without a crucifixion, no life without death; each element is a part of human reality related to our spiritual journey.

I believe in the probability of reincarnation. I live as if reincarnation is true. It helps me to be a better person, because I know if I am not virtuous I will reap the consequences— even in a future life. It makes sense to me that a loving God would allow us another chance to do it right, to make up for past mistakes. But I can't prove reincarnation. I don't believe that I am going to come back in this same body. But rather, the witness in me, the eye (I) watching me, experiencing my life and learning from it, will choose a new human form to return in, and learn some new lessons. Hopefully, it will be easier for me next time.

I believe life has many goals. I choose my goals, which teach me life's lessons, thus fulfilling my purpose. I believed I would eventually reach my goal of better health and improved physical functioning so long as I took each step necessary to complete the journey. I keep my end goal in mind so the process is just what I have to do, or go through, in order to get there.

I believe a primary purpose of life is to have fun. A key to my survival is my keen interest in what happens, good or bad, and my belief that everything that happens to me is an adventure. While going through many of these adventures, I may hate or fear them and wish I could avoid them.

I believe we must play life like a game. I'm still learning to do this. As a game it is fun, but when I play it for real, I often suffer. It's funny, because I don't like riding the roller coaster, which many people ride for excitement. But, I guess one could say the roller coasters I get my kicks from are some of the problems I've had in life. Sometimes I even think the more, the merrier. Just kidding! Cancel that potentially harmful seedthought!

I believe in taking myself seriously and also laughing at myself. I often told myself, "You are 'hot stuff' for having gone through brain surgery and surviving to report on it." Perhaps, at a subconscious level, the tumor and resultant surgery served to validate my whole existence.

I believe the mind is like a tape recorder. We have memory tapes which often get stuck, so we replay them over and over. Yet we can erase the pattern of memories being replayed with the tools I've written about. The content of the unconscious part of your mind often affects you as much as the content of your conscious mind and maybe even more. So it's important to get to know the hidden you and work to change any harmful unconscious programming.

I believe an important part of healing is learning to be comfortable with our emotions. The language of emotion is sparse, possibly a result of our difficulty handling emotions. Take the word "love." We have one word which we say to express the feeling of love for everything from food, to sex, to people. Surely we don't love each of these in the same way. We need new words to make distinctions between those different feelings of love. Learning to love and accept ourselves is basic to human education. So is learning to use language to express emotion in a positive way. Ultimately when we learn to truly love and accept ourselves, we'll be able to live well and love each other and every thing we encounter.

I believe in the power of affirmation, visualization, imagination, and prayer as tools for change. I use some of these techniques daily.

My first chosen affirmation, repeated over and over again early on in my quest to help my physical body, was, "I give thanks for my pure, perfect, whole, and holy body." A massage therapist I used then also kept telling me how healthy I was. At first I didn't believe it or her. My subconscious mind was invalidating the goal I was affirming by rebelling against the affirmation. Unhelpfully, I would say to myself, "Barbara, what makes you think you are healthy?"

But the therapist's positive belief about me and my practice affirmations worked well together. I soon realized that my body is a perfect vehicle for learning my life lessons, which made it easier to accept and give thanks for my perfect body. After a while I noticed how much better I was feeling. I found myself wholeheartedly affirming I was indeed healthy and had a body that worked very well.

I believe all healing ultimately stems from the mind and the Higher Power behind it. Sometimes we need to do something physical—like take medicine, or have surgery to support the mind's belief that healing will occur. We need external support because our minds aren't strong enough to believe the healing will occur without that physical aid. The mind alone, a gift from God, may well be able to heal any condition but for our disbelief. I wouldn't bet the farm on this one though—I'd go for expert medical advice.

I believe in the "law of agreement": an idea whose time has come depends on the agreement in principle of lots of people. Thoughts seem to get stronger the greater the number of people who believe in them. Many people agreed with me and told me they believed I would recover. That helped! Even now, whenever I am really worried, I may call a friend or other prayer partner. Each week I attend religious services during which I often pray for myself as well as others.

I believe in the power of religious affiliation and participation. Though I am Jewish, I wasn't always aware of the myriad ways my religion provides hope and healing prayer. I am now! Whenever I had a really tough experience to go through, I prayed, sometimes using the Twenty-Third Psalm and sometimes the Lord's Prayer, which I had memorized for just such tough times. At other times I inwardly chanted a mantra like "Om Namah Shivaya," or even made up an affirmation that was appropriate at the time. No matter what, I usually believed God was there with me, guiding my thoughts and actions. I felt that God was helping to heal me no matter which religion's rituals or prayers I was using. Today I mostly use Jewish prayers and rituals because I am now more comfortable with them.

I believe that I have a purpose—to be a translator and transformer. Transformers wake people up, helping to activate love, faith, forgiveness and service to the highest self. Translators speak the language of and see the good in others, be they different religions, or human potential and other groups that aren't religious, or even social movements like feminism. Different words often describe similar experiences and goals in or among different people. Translators help to synthesize divergent points of view by recognizing the common goals, purposes, and experiences of different people.

It may be easier to find fault rather than good in others, but it's not healing. There is power to heal ourselves and the planet in the concept of unity-in-diversity. That means we are one people, on planet Earth with many ways of expressing who we are and what and how we believe. But we are all connected and need one another to survive whether we are conscious of that fact or not.

***I believe in the power of forgiving.* Forgive and you shall be forgiven.**

I believe life is for-giving! I awakened my inner strength when I committed myself, many years ago, to the idea of being of service in the world. At that time, I became President of the Connecticut chapter of the National Organization for Women and started teaching and lecturing about "thinking for yourself."

I believe that "what goes around comes around." Life can either be like a vicious circle or a golden ring. "What you sow you reap." It's important for me to plant healthy seeds and to keep the soil of my life as weed-free, clear and fertile as possible. It's important for me to give, and then I feel worthy to receive.

I believe we can benefit from the experience of others. I expected people around me during my surgery and recovery period to benefit and get better as well. My attitude was, "If I have to suffer and go through difficulties like this, then at least other people should benefit making it more worthwhile for me." I was almost demanding that those around me improve themselves. Many did!

I believe in "making believe." I frequently made believe that I felt better than I really did. I pretended to everyone, sometimes even to myself. Pretending is the force that creates the new reality. Sometimes, I still pretend.

I believe ignorance is not bliss, because at some point we will wake up to the truth of reality. Sometimes I think I'd rather not be so aware. I don't want to know the future, but I'd still like to be prepared for different potential outcomes. I donít like being blind-sided or ambushed.

I seem to believe in "expect the best, prepare for the worst." I'm not yet sure whether that seedthought is good programming or not. Writing this book was often more uncomfortable than I expected. At times the only thing to do was to live through the discomfort, with as much non-judgmental awareness as I could muster. Often, after prayer, the problem cleared up just by living through it and observing it with detachment.

The past fifteen years have been a period of intense questioning for me as I reflect on my eleven-year quest to be free of the tumor. It is now thirty years since my first symptom— a paralyzed left vocal cord—led me in the right direction. I've explored the philosophies, the life and practices of different groups and religions, looking for healing alternatives. The tumor is gone, but my search continues for ways to heal the damage to my nerves. I am still learning, growing, asking questions, testing beliefs, loving the process. I used to live by "making the best of it." Now I believe in "making the most of it." There is a difference.

I believe that when we see our tough experiences from the perspective of distance in time, we often recognize them as blessings in disguise. At times, I asked myself, "If you know so much how come you couldn't heal yourself without surgery? How come it's taking so long to fully heal? Why do you still have physical limitations? Why did you have to go through all this?" But the answer came quickly, "Because going through all this taught you what you are sharing. Perhaps more importantly, your journey of tumor/growth/release allowed you the time and experiences you needed to change and improve yourself." The fact that things take time to resolve is truly the gift of time.

I believe that if we give people information and time, they will find truth. As Phil Donohue often said, "Let's hear some wisdom from the audience." Oprah Winfrey picked up where Donohue left off, respectfully trusting her audience to make good use of the information she and her guests shared with them.

I believe each person has the ability to think for themself and discern what's right for them.

I believe and trust in serendipity, those accidental (or maybe not so accidental) happenings in life that might actually be God working for our highest good. Watching televangelists on cable TV helped build my faith during the early stages of my healing. They propelled me to seek out a Rabbi who taught me what I hungered to learn and needed to know. I am grateful to those evangelists for their faith-filled preaching. I am especially thankful to my Rabbi who brought me back home to Judaism where I belong. It is said: "When the student is ready the teacher appears." That's true.

During the worst times, right after my brain surgery, when I was wheelchair-bound and unable to focus my eyes, I never lost hope. Deep inside, I always expected to get better. Prior to the surgery, I expected I'd be back to normal within a few months. I was really surprised by how physically damaged I was post-surgery. The degree of my difficulties caught me off guard, which could have easily led to despair. In fact, I had trouble even realizing what had happened to me. By the time it truly sank in how disabled I was, I had surrendered to the healing process. Some years later I recognized a seedthought "I was ambushed." I've changed the 'ambush' programming.

I see now that my faith was very deep. Given my prior emotional track record and my typical pattern of worrying, I could have been in a panic. But in fact, I was too busy doing what I could do, planning how to get well and following through, to spend time speculating that I might not recover. I used to think that I needed to worry in order to protect myself from some feared consequence or event. That belief has dissolved.

I believe in dwelling on best case, not worst case scenarios. Worry will not protect me from a disaster over which I have no control. If I feel a worry attack, where I am "awfulizing"—planting seedthoughts that say "this is awful"—by visualizing all kinds of unwanted occurrences, I turn to prayer or another activity to occupy my mind in a positive way. I use all the tools in this book and they help me.

It is my dream that each reader of this book will continue the journey within, arriving at better health and a richer, more rewarding life. It is my hope that each of you will think for your self—that inner Self—and recognize who and what that Self really is. It is my hope that you will be committed to your path, a peace-path, not a war-path, and that you will have faith that your journey through life will bring you the rewards you each deserve.

I believe you don't have to be sick to get better. It takes courage to live life fully, exploring and experiencing all that is there for you. I applaud your persistence, even as I have applauded my own.

My beliefs gave me the strength and will to survive the ordeal of brain surgery and the long recovery period. The more I understand who or what my Self really is, the more I believe in thinking for myself and in Self-induced healing.

Jewish mystics known as Kabbalists as well as mystics in many religious traditions point out that "the body is not the self. Since 'I' can speak of '*my* body' the body cannot be 'me.' The body is 'mine'—something associated with the 'me;' but the ultimate me is something much more profound than the body."[170]

Test the principles in this book in your own life. Use the exercises in this book to help you become more aware—of how you think, what you feel, and what you say. Recognize the creative power of your words and thoughts and see how they contribute to your version of life. Accept only that information which you know is for your highest good. Ignore what doesn't help you. Follow your intuition and your heart.

Self-Help Experience #50

Starting a Support Group—The Bliss Group

Purpose: To start a group to support people who are "okay" with themselves and who love life.

There are many groups that support people in times of trouble. Some are the anonymous groups like those serving alcoholics, drug addicts, child abuse victims, gamblers, etc. Others like ECAP (Exceptional Cancer Patients) serve those in a health crisis. Still other groups assist weight watchers or divorcees or widows. There seems to be a support group to help you through every kind of problem.

I believe everyone, in crisis or not, needs a loving support group. Social and religious organizations often provide this kind of support. I would encourage every reader to find a community of like-minded people to meet with for mutual support. I think one of the best places to find this nurturing is by partcipating in a social action or a religious communal group. Whether you join with others to serve your community or attend a synagogue, or church, or mosque, or ashram, you can find like-minded people to befriend and hang out with.

For a time, I was a member of a Bliss Group founded for the purpose of assisting each woman member in achieving a high-quality life and then spreading that good feeling to others. The key to the success of the participants in the Bliss Group was the affirmation each woman made in order to join: "I am the Source of life showing up as Bliss. I am committed to this women's group for one year." Thus, each woman was the source of, and responsible for, her group's success.

My Bliss Group met once a month in a different member's home. The hostess sent a letter to each member sharing her vision for the evening and choosing a topic she would like each of us to address. We had 16 women in our group. At one point there were about two hundred women committed to various Bliss Groups in a loosely structured network of women in New York and its suburbs who followed a monthly format similar to my group.

We had dinner, socialized, and usually spoke on a specific topic chosen in advance by the hostess of the evening. Two women served as resource for each group. My purpose as resource for my group was to assist the other members in whatever ways seemed appropriate to me. **Among the monthly discussions were some of the following topics:**

• How to achieve intimacy in relationships

• Loving ourselves and our bodies

• Managing money successfully

• Families: what are they, who are they?

• Friendships: meaning and purpose

• Integrity, trust, and authenticity

These were some sample visions for the evening's outcome:

• Each woman will feel closer to other members of the group.

• We will each be more responsible for ourselves and take better care of our bodies.

• We will improve our ability to handle money.

• We will each be more aware of and accepting of our own feelings, rather than the beliefs and feelings we adopted from others.

• Our friendships will be deeper, richer, and more mutually

Believe, when you are most unhappy, that there is something
for you to do in the world. So long as you can sweeten
another's pain, life is not in vain.
—Helen Keller

Self Help Experience # 51

Laughter As Medicine

Purpose: Finding and using your sense of humor. Everyone has one!

It's often been said that laughter is the best medicine. Laughter *is* contagious, infectious and good for your health whether you are sick or well.

Raising your laugh quotient requires a willingness to be open to perceiving what's so funny. Following are some time proven suggestions for increasing laughter in your life. If you expect to laugh you probably will.

Instructions:

Top 10 Things to Do to Improve Your Sense of Humor

1. Watch TV every day after telling yourself "I am watching TV for a humor break." Keep track of what strikes you as funny. You may have to watch several different kinds of shows before you find which ones tickle your funny bone.

2. Make use of your TV and VCR to keep a supply of laugh medicine on hand. There is comedy around the clock available on TV.

3. Watch video tapes of classic comedy shows as well as the latest favorites.

4. Watch TV comedians. You are likely to find some who can make you laugh.

5. You can keep your eyes closed, lie in bed, and still get a good laugh listening to comedy audio cassette tapes and compact discs.

6. Read the comics and cartoons in the newspaper.

7. Read books on humor such as *Compassionate Laughter: Jest for your Health* by Patty Wooten R.N.

8. Make use of e-mail and the Internet to find good humor sources.

9. Ask friends and family to share what they think is funny.

10. Look for the humor in your own life. Everyone can find something to laugh at.

Willingness is the key. For the best laugh of all, read the lists of how we talk at the end of Chapter 8.

Laughter is a tranquilizer with no side effects.
—Arnold Glasow

Self Help Experience #52

Prayers for Healing

Purpose: To experience the power of prayer in a context of interfaith understanding.

Perhaps these prayers have an intensified effect as a result of continuous usage. I remember once reading about a study where groups of people were taught rhymes from a foreign language. If the words used were from a popular nursery rhyme, the test subjects learned the words easier than they learned a new rhyme. It seems that the nursery rhyme was easier to learn, even though it was unfamiliar to the test subjects. Perhaps oft-repeated prayers, have some special power. As you read the prayers from religious traditions other than your own, remember that there are many paths leading to the same destination.

Jewish Prayer
Hear my voice, O Lord, when I call;
Be gracious to me and answer me. [Psalm 27:7]
In Thy hand is the soul of every living thing,
I turn to Thee, O Lord, in my distress.
Give me patience and faith;
Let not despair overwhelm me.
Renew my trust in Thy mercy
And bless the efforts of all who are helping me.

(continued) next page

Be with my dear ones in these difficult days.
Grant me Thy healing
So that in vigor of body and mind
I may return to my loved ones
For a life which will be marked by good deeds.

Catholic Prayer
Lord Jesus Christ,
you took our weakness on yourself
and bore our sufferings in your passion and death.
Hear this prayer for my suffering.
You are my redeemer:
strengthen my hope for salvation
and in your kindness sustain me in body and soul.
You live and reign for ever and ever. AMEN

Protestant Prayer
Gracious and merciful God,
because you have given your son,
I know that you are never far away from me.
I TURN TO YOU IN THIS quiet moment
to seek your comfort and strength.
Be my companion today, O Lord,
that I may receive your healing and renewing touch,
In Jesus' name, I pray. AMEN

Eastern Orthodox Prayer
O Holy Father, Physician of our souls and our bodies
Who sent Thine only begotten Son, our Lord Jesus Christ
Who has healed every disease and delivered us from death;
Heal me, Thy servant, through the grace of Thy Christ,
From the spiritual and physical infirmity which has come upon
    me.
And renew life in me according to Thy good pleasure, that
    owing Thee
Thanksgiving and worship, I may repay them in good works.

Hindu Prayer
You, O Lord, are the body's protector.
My body protect.
You, O Lord, are the giver of life.

Grant life to me.
From you, O Lord, comes brilliance of mind.
Illumine my mind.
Whatever is lacking to my being, O Lord, supply that to me.

Islamic Prayer
In the Name of God, the merciful Lord of mercy.
Praise be to God, the Lord of all being,
the merciful lord of mercy,
Master of the day of judgment.
You alone we serve; to You alone we come for aid.
Guide us in the straight path,
the path of those whom you have blessed,
not of those against whom there is displeasure,
nor of those who go astray.

Buddhist Prayer
Though I be suffering and weak, and all
My youthful spring be gone, yet have I come
Leaning upon my staff, and clambered up
The mountain peak.
My cloak thrown off,
My little bowl o'erturned, so I sit here
Upon the rock. And o'er my spirit sweeps
The breath of liberty! 'Tis won, 'tis won,
The Triple Lore! The Buddha's will is done.

Sufi Prayer
Beloved Lord,
Almighty God,
Through the rays of the sun,
Through the waves of the air,
Through the all pervading life in space;
purify and revivify me.
And I pray,
Heal my body, heart and soul.
AMEN.

More things are wrought by prayer than this world dreams of.
—Alfred, Lord Tennyson

Everything comes to a head.

The tide has turned.

Make the most of it.

Behind every dark cloud there is a rainbow.

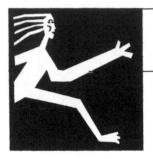

January, 2000

Epilog

In the spring of 1988, I began the final editing of the first edition of this book under the guidance of my then publisher, Dawson Church. Part of the task was to include some of the latest research, especially related to the immune system. Since I originally finished that manuscript, many books and articles had appeared that supported what I had written. Final editing and research was engrossing. Although I'd never before written under such a tight deadline, I joyfully welcomed the opportunity to complete my book's gestation and give birth to it.

I've been told that in writing a book and sharing one's own personal growth, a person often finds unfinished business "coming to a head." Problem areas can be faced, the experience digested, and the author is then released to grow into the next challenging space in her life. For example, when I finished the initial draft of the first edition back in 1984, I found that I still had a brain tumor which had actually become life threatening. I had surgery and that rare growth was released.

Still, I was surprised by what happened as I finished the final draft of the first edition in 1989. I had been feeling very strong and healthy. But I was "stewing" emotionally over difficulties involving a family-owned business run by my husband.

On May 3, 1989 (my daughter Jennifer's 19th birthday), I had a magnetic resonance imaging (MRI) exam of my brain. I thought it would be a routine follow-up exam—as if an MRI or CAT scan can ever be considered routine. It was then an integral part of my yearly checkup to ensure that I remained tumor free.

On May 4, I was told that something unforeseen was discovered. I spent a somewhat restless night. For me, I was really quite calm. Not knowing what to think, I prayed a lot.

On May 5, Dr. Lipow, a neurosurgeon, showed me the MRI pictures. I saw what appeared to be a rather large growth in my skull. I felt like I was back in an old nightmare, only this time I might not wake up. From the size of this *thing*, and the speed of its growth from nothing there the year before, it looked ominous. The doctor said it could be anything from virulent cancer to scar tissue, to an infection from some unknown source. The latter seemed a likely diagnosis since I had had a left ear infection in March and my ear had begun draining again several weeks prior to the MRI.

I felt a combination of hope, fear, unbelief, and anger. I felt betrayed, by what or whom I didn't identify. Though I surely had the strength and the will to live, I was very clear that I didn't want to go on another brain tumor/surgery trip. I wanted time to finish my book, but when thinking of the worst case possibilities—brain surgery, brain cancer, chemotherapy—I didn't want to live. My sense of being ambushed by fate was very strong.

Strangely, despite my upset, and despite the evidence, I didn't really believe what was happening. I mean, the evidence was before me, I was taking it seriously, but in many ways, it just wasn't real to me. I vowed to go through this with faith, not fear. Deep inside me, I expected to be okay.

On Monday, May 7— in order to see if there was an extra-large blood supply to this *thing* which would indicate that it was a solid or malignant tumor— I had an arteriogram. That meant a hospital stay and the repeat of an unpleasant procedure which I still remembered from years before.

The next day Dr. Lipow gave me the good news, there was no extra blood supply to my *thing*, so it was unlikely to be a tumor. He suspected an abscess and said I'd need surgery that week to remove it.

I wanted to wait till I finished revising the book, but Dr. Lipow didn't think that was wise or safe. However, before setting a definite date for surgery, he was waiting for the report from the hospital's infectious disease department to see if the blood work etc. showed any signs of acute infection throughout my body.

I decided to play it positively and took a walk through the hospital halls, praising and thanking God for healing me. I put no conditions on the healing, I just acted and thought positively. Within the hour word came that I had no sign of infection anywhere else in my body. If the thing on the MRI was an infection, it was localized and not threatening my life. At that point, the doctor said we could wait and first try a more conservative treatment of antibiotics. Then I would be X-rayed again to see if the thing was gone. I was thrilled that I would have the time to complete my research and finish writing the book.

I am amazed at how calm I was over the next few weeks. I immersed myself in reading articles in journals and books with case studies that related to immune function and other pertinent topics— becoming more convinced than ever that the mind can cure the body. The fruits of that work are scattered throughout the book. My prayers were for a perfect healing for myself.

I discovered a primary seedthought. I was "stewing" over my husband's business problems and heard myself say, "When the (business) crisis came to a head, my new growth was discovered." One day, as I wrote a history of my husband's business problems, the connection between the two seemed stronger than ever. As I wrote, my ear kept oozing, at a faster rate than at any other time that month. It seems like my emotions connected to my husband's troubles were "stewing around in my head."

On June 3, I went for a CAT scan, filled with hope that all signs of the *thing*, as I called it, would be gone and I wouldn't need surgery. The ear drainage had stopped the week before. But immediately after the CAT scan, the drainage began again, and I felt hopeless.

On June 5, I got the result. There was no change from the previous month. The only way to know for sure what was wrong was an operation to go in and look. I still remember thinking: "I should be able to heal myself." The alternative— another operation, a biopsy—was appalling to me.

I had begun to hear criticism of the holistic health movement because people read books by Louise Hay, Bernie Siegel or other best-selling authors, used the techniques and they didn't seem to work. The patient was still sick or even sicker and felt angry and ripped off. Now, I was facing these same feelings and I had written the book.

I understood first-hand how people sometimes feel when they find they haven't cured themselves of some physical problem. I felt like a failure! Despite my belief that the process is as important as the end result (in terms of personal growth and learning), I still felt enormous guilt. "Why couldn't I, of all people (with all my knowledge and self-help practice), cure myself without drugs or surgery?"

I realized rather quickly that a perfect healing didn't necessarily mean I would be able to avoid surgery. A perfect healing, for me, might involve knowing for sure what caused the *thing* on the X-ray. A perfect healing for me might be to face my fears, have the surgery, and come through easily. I recognized immediately that one of my biggest fears was "being ambushed," "being caught by surprise," "being unprepared."

One part of me expected the best, but a deeper part feared the worst—no wonder I tended to worry about everything and to rehearse all kinds of negative scenarios. Now I had a chance to heal that tendency and change the seedthoughts feeding my unhealthy core belief. Back then I had a core belief that imagining the worst would protect me from the worst. But actually given what I know about the power of imagination, pretending the worst seems more like praying for the wrong thing than getting prepared for the worst.

I recognized that I often went to the doctor in hopes of being reassured that I was okay, not really to find a cure for what ailed me. Then, when the doctor did find something wrong (even if it was curable), I often felt ambushed. I eventually realized that it *is* possible to expect the best and still be prepared if the worst happens. Besides, the worst case scenario rarely happens.

For a month I kept working, finishing the first edition of *Your Body Believes Every Word You Say* on July 2, 1989. All the while I used some natural therapies and prayers to improve my health and prepare myself for the inevitable operation. I hoped that the biopsy would show I had a cyst which could be drained easily and I would be done with it. I released my guilt and felt quite certain that what I was going through was the epilog to the book. Somehow, this experience would tie everything I'd learned together.

On July 5, 1989, I had surgery, which was much easier than I expected— I was home the next day. There was no tumor! The surprise diagnosis was a chronic mastoid infection. The mastoid bone looked like a congested beehive. Just about every cell in the mastoid was filled with infection. Dr. Gill, the ear surgeon, was surprised at how extensive it was, considering that I had had only one symptomatic ear infection in the previous six months.

While I was enormously relieved that the tumor had not recurred, at first I felt dismay at the thought of many more months of antibiotic treatment. Evidence of how I dealt with this was my comment to friends, "Antibiotics (a biochemical therapy for infection) sure beats my needing chemotherapy for cancer." After several days, I made peace with the therapy and developed a genuine attitude of gratitude at how lucky I was. I had never been one to want to "take a pill to get well," but I hoped it would work this time.

A year of antibiotic therapy caused no discomfort. I kept my body well nourished throughout with friendly intestinal flora and other immune system boosters. The ear drainage ceased after a few months. Then a 1990 MRI brain scan showed improvement from the previous year.

I joyfully received my perfect healing as I recognized that getting rid of an illness, while desirable, really is only a part of the healing process—loving and accepting oneself is as important. Getting rid of fear and releasing the past completes the process. Being able to enjoy life, no matter what, is key.

Learning from everything that happens *is* healthy behavior. I became more adept at harmonizing my emotions and releasing those worries about which I could do nothing. The problems related to my husband's business back then were resolved, and I felt happier and healthier than I had in years.

In November 1990, the first copy of *Your Body Believes Every Word You Say: The Language of the Body/Mind Connection* arrived in my home. I felt gratitude, awe, humility and pride. Doing what I could to promote the book, I enjoyed the sense of freedom that comes with completion of a long worked on task.

I soon became aware of a deep spiritual hunger and a need to explore Judaism, my birth religion, as a faith and a way of life. The journey profoundly influenced my life and work on this book.

In 1993, after learning to chant Hebrew from the Torah—a sacred scroll containing the first five books of the Bible—I chanted before the Congregation and celebrated my Bat Mitzvah. In the process of preparing and accomplishing this, I recognized and released many core beliefs about my disabilities that had been preventing me from fully savoring my life. I began to relish just being alive, no matter what, as I learned to live in a deeply satisfying new way, in harmony with the Jewish calendar, which is a lunar calendar.

In 1994 my original publisher first approached me about doing an updated second edition of *Your Body Believes Every Word You Say*. I began saving information to add to a new version. I told myself and everyone else that I was working on a new edition, but I was *not* actually writing. There were myriad ways I procrastinated, sometimes by inadvertently feeding myself negative seedthoughts.

In the spring of 1996, I became very conscious of the passing of time and my need to make each day count while performing the annual Jewish ritual called "Counting the Omer." During this ritual, one counts and blesses each day with a special prayer for 49 days between the Jewish festivals of Passover and Shavuot. Passover celebrates the Jews exodus from Egypt and Shavuot commemorates the day at Sinai we received the Torah which includes the 10 Commandments.

I recognized more clearly than ever that human life is a journey, death the final destination and in between is the time we have to spend and what we do with that time. My focus on the importance of using my time wisely played a pivotal role in what happened when I finally began writing this revised and updated edition of *Your Body Believes Every Word You Say*.

In October 1996, after months of procrastination, I began to *really* write. But still I got precious little done as my life was filled with distractions.

By December 1996, things began falling into place after I finally committed myself to writing full time. But as long as we live, fresh challenges and new opportunities for growth will arise. Later that month, I faced a new challenge that would soon reach near crisis proportions.

Everything related to the writing seemed to work easily, if

not effortlessly. I was working very hard. However, every time I needed a study, a quote, some new information, it appeared as if by magic in a print article, on TV, or on the Internet—too often to be mere coincidence. I was generally awestruck at my good fortune, which can feel so good and so awful both at the same time. Good because when life flows so easily and effort-lessly—I feel in control. Awful because I know that I am not in control of everything that happens—only of my attitude about what happens.

I was pre-occupied with the idea of spending time fruitfully and not wasting time. Underneath these thoughts was my fear that, like my parents so many years ago, I might die sooner rather than later. Adding fuel to my fear of aging and early death were the unexpected deaths of two friends and a dear cousin—all about my age.

I began to worry that I was going to die before doing the things I still wanted to do such as completing the books I wanted to write. A new seedthought *"not enough time"* was having a negative effect on me emotionally even while providing me with a strong incentive to write each day and get it done.

On December 23— with work on the first draft of this edition of the book going extremely well—I thought that per-haps after all, "there would be enough time to get the work done." Wondering "How come I am so lucky?" and "Why me?" I inexplicably began crying. Giving thanks for the bless-ings I was receiving, I was at the same time praying that I would live long enough to enjoy any success coming my way.

I suddenly felt extremely, unbearably frightened that I might soon die. I had no clue back then as to what triggered this intense emotion.

Since it was after 10 p.m. on the East Coast when I felt the most frightened, I called my friend and spiritual teacher Rabbi Ted Falcon in Seattle, where it was only 7 p.m. In addition to leading a Congregation, he is an author, meditation teacher and psychotherapist. I trusted him to understand what I was going through and to share words of wisdom. By the time I spoke to him, I was able to unemotionally report my feelings. Looking back, I had actually gone numb.

Rabbi Falcon felt that what I was going through was clearly related to my work on the book. I was surprised when he said, "It's necessary for you to add something that was missing in the first edition." He then advised me to "face my shadow." I didn't know what he meant, nor how to achieve it.

I did know that my writing tends to release suppressed emotion—then I can write from a point of personal understanding. I recognized that this would most likely make me feel uncomfortable, but I knew that there was nothing I could do short of aborting the whole process. Quitting was not an option. Since I was eager to finally write this new edition, I knew I would go through with the process, like it or not.

After speaking with Rabbi Falcon, I wondered about my shadow and decided he was referring to the numerous negative things I was thinking and feeling. I believe it was the knowledge that such negative thoughts were even there, lurking in my mind, that had made me feel so upset. I was afraid those seedthoughts and feelings were gaining a foothold, preventing me from being positive and upbeat. And knowing what I know of the power of seedthoughts, I was scared of the impact that such thoughts would have on me physically as well as emotionally.

There were many mixed blessings in my life. For example, in 1995, I went from an empty nest and being alone much of the time to a full house. My son, his wife and their two daughters—our precious grandchildren—had come to live with us. This provided good company and positive bonding opportunities with them among other gifts, at the price of a neat house, space, freedom and privacy.

At first, those impediments had seemed of little import. But after two years I was feeling trapped by this family situation which, at first, had brought me joy and comfort. By then I felt as if I couldn't stand it another minute. I felt like I had no space of my own in which to breathe. And no change was possible for some time because the time was not yet ripe for them to move out.

There were other troubling situations adding to the chaos and uncertainty I was experiencing. One involved money. Another concern was who would actually be publishing this book when I completed revising and updating it since the original Aslan Publishing company was for sale and still held the publishing rights. In the process of living my life, along with the many blessings, I had my inevitable share of trials and tribulations. It often seemed to me that many of the good things in my life carried a price that was hard for me to pay.

I had begun complaining because the rose bush had thorns rather than rejoicing because the thorn bush had roses. I judged myself harshly for even daring to complain. My operative seedthought was, "There is always someone worse off than you." I was feeling guilty and depressed coming face to face with my shadow.

Early in February 1997, I told my friend author Steven Rosman how guilty I felt for complaining when I was really so blessed. His response startled me, "Barbara, you are being too hard on yourself and burdening yourself unnecessarily." I had always believed that other people were too self-judgmental or critical of themselves but that I was actually too easy on myself. I had never thought that I was too hard on myself. *"Could it be true?"*

Later that week, I met with my Rabbi, Jim Prosnit, telling myself beforehand, "I will feel better if I talk to him." I didn't even realize at the time that I had planted a useful seedthought in my mind. After the meeting I thought, "I'm really not so bad." Rabbi Prosnit had reminded me that I am a capable, loving person who cares about doing good in the world. I felt better, although that day I was still not quite my formerly sunny and positive thinking self.

However, by **the following Saturday, February 8**, after synagogue services, I felt happier than I had in a long time. I had begun to release my negative self judgments. I was moving from despair to hope, from negative thinking to a more positive outlook, from hiding in the shadows to rejoicing in the light. I remember thinking, "*the worst is over, now I will be okay.*"

But the weeks of negative thinking and upset, added to the stress and pressure in my life circumstances, had taken a toll. There was still lots more emotion and other things to "get off my chest."

That afternoon, I began coughing up blood.

Several years earlier, I had coughed blood for one month before finally receiving an accurate diagnosis of a lung abscess, which led to proper treatment with intravenous antibiotics and a cure after a week in the hospital. Because of neurological damage resulting from the brain tumor, I have a tendency to aspirate and therefore I am at greater risk of such lung infections. Fortunately, I'd only been ill that one time, perhaps due to what I still believe is my strong immune system.

So it was an unexpected shock to again cough up blood. From past experience and after consultation with several physicians, I knew this illness was not a life-threatening emergency, so I felt safe waiting a few days to see pulmonary specialist Dr. David Bushell. But I was annoyed that my life was being interrupted again by a reaction in my body. I didn't have time to be sick or hospitalized.

Dr. Bushell's examination and a chest X-ray proved negative. A CAT scan was scheduled for that **Wednesday, February 12** in order to rule out anything hidden behind the scar tissue from the prior lung abscess. If Dr. Bushell was looking for anything more ominous he did not tell me. Actually, he wisely re-assured me that it was entirely possible that this "coughing blood" episode was a benign one that would correct itself without any treatment. Though I wanted to believe him, I still had doubts.

I prayed for a sign to reassure me. Shortly thereafter, Jessica Rosenblatt, a Hebrew school teacher friend, told me about someone she knew who'd had a similar experience which turned out to be self-limiting and of no consequence. Jessica's words answered my prayer—God *was* with me. Still I had to go through the whole process, deal with the cause of the bleeding, and rule out whatever.

The next day I learned that the CAT scan was negative. There was no change from the baseline CAT scan done after my lung abscess episode in 1995. No further tests, nor any treatment, were required. Within a week, I stopped coughing blood. During this entire episode my husband and family were incredibly supportive and reassuring. I kept working on the book and made extensive progress.

Shortly thereafter, I first recognized that when I began dealing with a physical condition, the self-pity about my life circumstances and accompanying negative thoughts and depressed feelings left me. The physical problems banished the emotional and spiritual ones from my mind.

In retrospect, I realize that I actually began feeling better emotionally just before the emotional upsets from my spiritual malaise manifested as a physical problem. I had even begun to enjoy having the family live with us. Even though the circumstances in my life hadn't yet changed, as I faced my shadow self I changed, so everything in my life seemed different and I felt better.

There must be something to the notion that we often transmit our subconscious feelings even when we try to hide them, because my granddaughters began responding to me more positively than they had in a while.

By March 1997, I had finally recognized and understood the core belief fueling my fears and my tears that night back in December 1996 when I had been so terrified. Although then my work was going very well, I feared that I wouldn't live long enough to enjoy the fruits of my labor. I thought that I really had no control. Later I realized that a powerful seedthought which had undermined me was "I don't *deserve* such good treatment or to be so blessed."

I saw that I was unwittingly feeding myself a lot of negative thoughts, never allowing myself to be truly satisfied, nor giving myself enough credit for what I was accomplishing. I *was* being too hard on myself. This has now been replaced by a healthier belief system. I am not so hard on myself anymore because I feel worthy of the blessings I receive.

Now, I appreciate how much I am accomplishing each day even if I don't get everything done. Instead of berating myself as a master procrastinator, I remind myself that I am taking my time to really prepare the ground for future growth, accomplishment and prosperity. I often acknowledge how much fun I am having in the process.

I realize too that just because I am better off than someone else doesn't mean I have no right to complain. It's useless to compare myself to others either favorably or unfavorably. I am who I am and my life is *my* life. Perhaps acknowledging the strengthening and renewal of my faith in myself and in God is the key to fully understanding my experience.

Since the above episode early in 1997, a lot has changed and is still changing. In October of that year, shortly after I began noticing the roses more often than the thorns, my husband and I became the owners of Aslan Publishing, regaining control of the publishing rights to this book. I love being a publisher and creative director and am still filled with immense gratitude at this unexpected turn of events. And even without the positive feedback I receive, I know I am good at my job. Now I know who will be publishing this book. :-)

Furthermore, **in August 1999**, my son and his family moved out of our house. Finally the time was ripe, everything worked out for the best and we accomplished even more than the goals we hoped to achieve when they first began living with us. They are happy and we are happy.

I firmly believe that life always works out for my benefit and my highest good. I sometimes will still question whether I am using my time wisely, but I now know that even so-called wasted time counts, especially if I don't judge myself so harshly and instead choose to enjoy each moment. Also, worrying about time or anything else will not ensure a better future and might actually make things worse for a while.

There may still be buttons in me to be pressed, raw spots that need healing, but I will deal creatively with them. To be a healthy human being means that one will always have lessons to learn, challenges to face, problems to deal with, new opportunities for growth, and unconscious shadows to be brought into the light.

Life may well be a journey with death the final destination, but it *is* meant to be lived as best as we can, as long as we can, no matter what. Living life, getting to know oneself, uncovering core beliefs, uprooting negative seedthoughts and planting healthy new ones is truly a life-long, never-ending process.

As I complete writing this epilog, it is nearly 30 years since my left vocal cord was first paralyzed. With joy, I share the second edition of *Your Body Believes Every Word You Say.* Having written it, I understand more about myself, others, psychology, spirituality and health. I also have more faith in my ability and God's willingness to provide for me.

Though from time to time I forget, I know that I AM both the observer and the observed, the thoughts and the actions, the words and the deeds, the Creator and the Created. I AM the process of my life. This knowing led to my healing, my mission in life and this book, my bequest to the world.

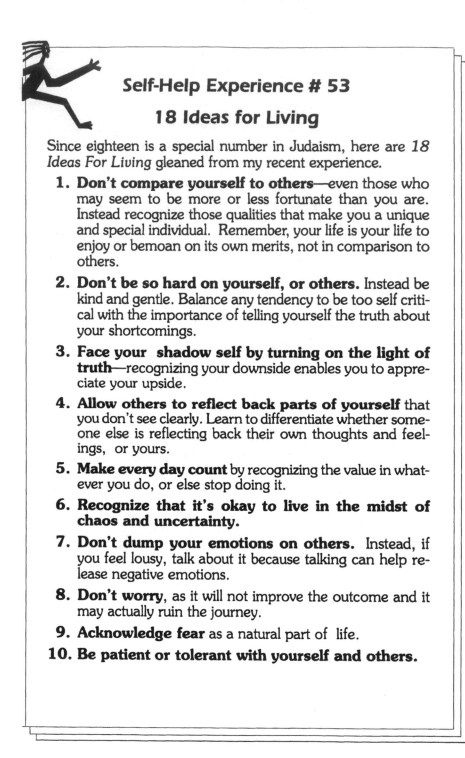

Self-Help Experience # 53

18 Ideas for Living

Since eighteen is a special number in Judaism, here are *18 Ideas For Living* gleaned from my recent experience.

1. **Don't compare yourself to others**—even those who may seem to be more or less fortunate than you are. Instead recognize those qualities that make you a unique and special individual. Remember, your life is your life to enjoy or bemoan on its own merits, not in comparison to others.

2. **Don't be so hard on yourself, or others.** Instead be kind and gentle. Balance any tendency to be too self critical with the importance of telling yourself the truth about your shortcomings.

3. **Face your shadow self by turning on the light of truth**—recognizing your downside enables you to appreciate your upside.

4. **Allow others to reflect back parts of yourself** that you don't see clearly. Learn to differentiate whether someone else is reflecting back their own thoughts and feelings, or yours.

5. **Make every day count** by recognizing the value in whatever you do, or else stop doing it.

6. **Recognize that it's okay to live in the midst of chaos and uncertainty.**

7. **Don't dump your emotions on others.** Instead, if you feel lousy, talk about it because talking can help release negative emotions.

8. **Don't worry**, as it will not improve the outcome and it may actually ruin the journey.

9. **Acknowledge fear** as a natural part of life.

10. **Be patient or tolerant with yourself and others.**

11. **Learn to wait patiently**. Remember Ecclesiastes "A season is set for everything, a time for every experience under heaven."

12. **Learn when to trust and follow the inner wisdom that is your intuition** and when to give up control over life to a Higher Power. Spend some quiet time each day listening carefully to that "still small voice."

13. **Remember God is on your side** and wants you to be happy.

14. **Rejoice in life's blessings** rather than dwell on the negatives.

15. **Be careful what you wish for**—you just might get it.

16. **Think of the journey through life as a roller coaster ride**—sometimes you are up, feeling on top of the world— and at other times you are speeding downhill seemingly out of control.

17. **Recognize the importance of putting a proper "spin" on an experience** because it is not so much what happens to us that helps or hurts—it is what we tell ourselves about what happens that determines its effect on us.

18. **Remember that death is inevitable for us all but life is meant to be lived fully until our last day.** We may each be on a terminal path but we can remain more, or less, healthy throughout our journey until we reach the terminal that is...

The End

End Notes

Chapter 2

1. from a personal conversation with Dr. Schweitzer in 1989.
2. from a personal conversation with Dr. Sica in 1997.
3. Joan Borysenko, *Minding The Body, Mending The Mind*, New York: Bantam Books, 1988, p. 13.
4. ibid. p. 14.
5. ibid. p. 15.
6. ibid. p. 16.
7. ibid. p. 16.
8. from a phone conversation with Dr. Randall Neichen in 1997.
9. Norman Cousins in an excerpt from *JAMA*, Sept. 16, 1988, Vol. 260 #11, reprinted in *Noetic Sciences Review*, Winter 1988.
10. Tom Monte et. al.,*World Medicine: The East-West Guide to Healing Your Body* , New York: GP Putnam's Sons, 1993, pg. 294.
11. Institute of HeartMath, 14700 West Park Ave., Boulder Creek, CA 95006, 831-338-8700 / 831-338-9861 fax
    Website: www.heartmath.org/ Email: hrtmath@netcom.com
12. ibid., "The Effects of Emotions on Short Term Heart Rate Variability Using Power Spectrum Analysis," *American Journal of Cardiology*, November 15, 1995, pages 1089-93.
13. For more information on this study, along with a description of the technique used in the research, refer to: "CUT-THRU," by Doc Lew Childre, Planetary Publications,1996.
14. Andy Geller, *New York Post*, Nov. 16, 1996.
15. ibid.
16. ibid.
17. Howard and Martha Lewis, *Psychosomatics: How Your Emotions Can Damage Your Health*, New York: Viking Press, 1972, p. 10.
18. Ronald Glasser, M.D., *The Body Is the Hero*, New York: Random House, 1976, p. 228-9.
19. Buryl Payne, "A Theory of Mind: How We Create Our Reality," (unpublished article, 1984).
20. Bette Runck from world net article, U.S. Department of Health and Human Services DHHS Publication No. (ADM) 83-1273, 1983.
21. Norman Cousins, *The Healing Heart*, New York: Norton & Co. 1893, p. 200-01.
22. ibid. p. 202.
23. James J. Lynch, *The Broken Heart: The Medical Consequences of Loneliness*, New York: Basic Books 1977, cover flap.
24. Andrew Weil, M.D., is the author of numerous books including *Spontaneous Healing: How to Discover and Enhance Your Body's Natural Ability to Maintain and Heal Itself*, Ballantine Books, 1996, and *Natural Health, Natural Medicine*, Houghton-Mifflin, 1995.
25. from a conversation in 1997 with CPA Steven Levine, then a senior manager with Price-Waterhouse.
26. K. J. Petrie, D. Buick and J. Weinman, "Positive Effects of Illness Reported by Myocardial Infarction and Breast Cancer Patients" (abstract), *Psychosomatic Medicine* 1996; Vol. 58, #76. Cited in *Mind/Body Health* newsletter, 1996, Vol. V #2.

27. Paul Pearsall, Ph.D., *Superimmunity: Master Your Emotions and Improve Your Health*, New York: McGraw-Hill, 1987, p. 112.
28. ibid.
29. "Mental Control of Immune Function," *Mental Medicine Update* Fall 1993, pg. 7.

Chapter 3
30. James W. Lance, *Headache:Understanding Alleviation*, New York: Scribners, 1975, p. 92.
31. Carolyn Reuben, "AIDS: The Promise of Alternative Treatments," *East-West Journal*, Sept. 1986, p. 52-66.
32. Andrew Sullivan, "When Plagues End," *New York Times Magazine*, Nov.10, 1996, p. 54.
33. from a personal interview with Dr. Ron Levin in February, 1997.
34. Paul Pearsall, *Super Immunity*, p. 319.
35. During a personal interview with Bear in 1983.
36. "Mind/ Hypertension Link,"*Brain/Mind Bulletin,* July 1989, p. 2. A review of an article in the *Journal of Nervous and Mental Disease*, Vol. 177, p. 15-24, by John Sommers-Flanagan and Roger Greenberg.
37. from a personal conversation with Dr. Kunkes in December, 1996.
38. Thomas Pickering, M.D., *Socioeconomic Determinants of Hypertension and Its Control*, an address delivered to the American Society of Hypertension, 10th Annual Scientific Meeting, May 18, 1995. (reprinted on the Internet).
39. from a personal interview with Dr. Sica in March, 1997.
40. from a personal interview with Dr. Bushell in February, 1997.
41. *The Living Bible*, James 3:3-7.
42. Rabbi Stephen M. Wylen, "Midrash Sohar tov 120," *Gossip: The Power of the Word*, KTAV Publishing House, 1993, p. 149.
43. from personal private correspondence.

Chapter 4
44. Viktor E. Frankl, M.D., Ph.D., *Man's Search For Meaning: An Introduction to Logotherapy*, Boston: Beacon Press, 1962, p. 65-6.
45. W. C. Ellerbroek, M.D., "Language, Thought and Disease," *Co-Evolution Quarterly*, Spring, 1978, #17, p. 37.
46. from phone interviews with Dr. Ellerbroek in 1983.
47. Warren Berland, Ph.D., "Can the Self Affect the Course of Cancer?" *ADVANCES: The Journal of Mind-Body Health*, Fall 1995, Vol. 11 #4, p. 5-19.
48. ibid.
49. "Experts, Survivors Offer Hope At AIDS Meeting" and "Survivors Beating Odds with Belief, Humor and Self-reliance," *Brain/Mind Bulletin*, March 1989, Vol. 14, #6.
50. Mark Schoofs, "The Berlin Patient" in *New York Times Magazine*, June 21, 1998, p. 34.
51. Ronald J. Glasser, M.D., *The Body Is the Hero*, back cover.
52. Dennis T. Jaffe, *Healing From Within*, New York: Alfred Knopf, 1980, p.121.
53. ibid., p. 122-3, reporting on a study by W. J. Grace and D. T. Graham: "Relationship of Specific Attitudes and Emotions to Certain Bodily Diseases," *Psychosomatic Medicine*, 1952, Vol.14, p. 243-51.
54. Milton Ward, *The Brilliant Function of Pain*, Lakemont, Georgia: CSA Press, 1977, p. 13.

55. from personal conversations in 1984.

Chapter 5
56. from a personal interview with Graham in 1984.
57. Viktor E. Frankl, *Man's Search For Meaning: An Introduction to Logotherapy*, p. 124.
58. ibid.

Chapter 6
59. from a personal interview with Marshall in 1984.
60. Tony Schwartz, "Doctor Love," *New York Magazine*, June 12, 1989, p. 42.
61. James J. Lynch, *The Broken Heart*, p. 57.
62. Personal email correspondence, 12/6/96.
63. Janice K. Kiecolt-Glaser and Ronald Glaser, "Psychological Influences on Immunity: Implications for Aids," *American Psychologist*, 1988; Vol. 43, #11, p. 892-898.
64. Paul Pearsall, *Super Immunity*, p. 7.
65. ibid. p. 9-10.
66. Barbara B. Brown, Ph.D., *Super Mind: The Ultimate Energy*, New York: Harper & Row, 1980, p. 30-31.

Chapter 7
67. From a personal interview with Alice Katz in 1988.
68. *Brain/Mind Bulletin*, April, 1989, p. 3.
69. Bernie Siegel, M.D., *Love, Medicine & Miracles*, New York: Harper & Row, 1986, p. 32.
70. during a healing panel meeting at Congregation Beth El in Fairfield CT, March, 1997.
71. From a personal interview with Bondi in 1984.

Chapter 8
72. from a personal interview with Zelizer in 1984.
73. from a personal interview with Dr. Kunkes in 1984.
74. from a personal interview with Dr. Ruzga in 1984.
75. from personal interviews in 1996-97 with Richard Levin, M.D., Ken Sacks, M.D., and Robert Burd, M.D., among other doctors mentioned throughout this book.
76. from a phone conversation with Dr. Lang in 1984.
77. from personal interviews with Hirshorn in 1997.
78. from several personal interviews with Tager in 1984.
79. from a personal interview with Dr. Scavo in 1984.
80. from a personal interview with Dr. Bushell in 1997.
81. from a personal interview with Dr. Hirshorn in 1997.
82. from a personal interview with Zelizer in 1984.
83. from a personal interview with Dr. Gruning in 1984.
84. from a fundraising letter during the 1980's.
85. William Safire, *New York Times,* Magazine Section, May 4, 1997, P. 22.
86. ibid.
87. from an interview with Tager in 1984.

Chapter 9
88. speaking at a Congregation B'nai Israel Religious School Assembly, Jan. 1995.
89. Daniel Goleman, Ph.D., *Vital Lies, Simple Truths: The Psychology of Self-Deception*, New York: Simon and Schuster, 1985, p. 90.
90. from Edgar Cayce literature obained from the A.R.E. Foundation.
91. Paul Pearsall, *Super Immunity*, p. 19.
92. ibid. p. 19-20.
93. from personal interviews with Tager in 1984.
94. George F. Solomon, M.D., "The Emerging Field of Psychoneuroimmunology" *Advances: The Journal For Mind-Body Health,* Institute for the Advancement of Health, Vol. 2 #1, p. 8.
95. ibid.
96. during personal interviews with Zelizer in 1983-84.

Chapter 10
97. During a workshop led by Dr. Bernie Siegel in Connecticut, 1988.
98. Norman Cousins, *The Healing Heart*, p. 204.
99. During a personal interview with Dr. Ruzga in 1984.
100. Bernie S. Siegel, *Love, Medicine & Miracles*, p. 47.
101. Daniel Goleman, *Vital Lies, Simple Truths*, p. 89-90.
102. during a personal interview with Tager in 1984.
103. during personal interviews with Esselstyn in 1984.
104. Sheryl Gay Stolberg, "Sham Surgery Returns as a Research Tool," New York Times, Sunday, April 25, 1999.
105. from an article by psychologist Bruno Klopfer, "Psychological Variables in Human Cancer," *Journal of Projective Techniques*, 1957, Vol 21, p. 329-340.
106. Ronald J. Glasser, *The Body Is The Hero*, p. 230-237.
107. Caryle Hirshberg and Marc Ian Barasch, *Remarkable Recoveries: What Extraordinary Healings Tell Us About Getting Well and Staying Well*, New York: Riverhead Books, 1995, p. 172-3 & p. 347.
108. ibid.
109. ibid. p. 173-4.
110. John Bradshaw, "Cradle Hypnosis," program #14 in the television series *The Eight Stages of Man*, Public Broadcasting System (PBS), 1989.
111. Paul Pearsall, *Superimmunity*, p. 10.
112. David Van Biema, "Learning to Live with a Past That Failed," *People Magazine*, May 29, 1989, p. 79-92. Cover article note, p. 4.
113. Dr. Bernard Lown, introduction to Cousins, *The Healing Heart*, p. 13-16.
114. Hirshberg & Barasch, *Remarkable Recoveries: What Extraordinary Healings Tell Us About Getting Well and Staying Well*, foreward, p. xiii.
115. ibid. p. xiv.

Chapter 11
116. Stephen S. Hall, "A Molecular Code Links Emotions, Mind and Health," *Smithsonian*, June 1989, p. 62-71.
117. ibid. p. 64.
118. The Kripalu Experience Program Guide, April-Sept. 1988, p. 21.
119. Tristine Rainer, *The New Diary*, Los Angeles: J. P. Tarcher, 1978, p. 138.

Chapter 12
120. *Brain/Mind Bulletin*, 1979, Vol IV # 5.
121. *Brain/Mind Bulletin*, 1977-8, Vol III #7.
122. *Brain/Mind Bulletin*, 1977, Vol. I #21, quoting Larry Siegel and William Fleeson of the Institute for Social Rehabilitation, and Alan Abrams of Far West Laboratories in San Francisco.
123. *Brain/Mind Bulletin*, 1977-8, Vol. III #18, a study conducted by dream researcher Henry Reed from *Journal of Clinical Psychology*, Vol. 34 #1, p. 150-158.
124. *Brain/Mind Bulletin*, 1980, Vol. V #4.
125. *Brain/Mind Bulletin*, Vol. II #14, summarizing an article in *New England Journal of Medicine*, Vol. 294 #2, p. 80-84.
126. *Brain/Mind Bulletin*, 1977, Vol. I #21, quoting Larry Siegel and William Fleeson of the Institute for Social Rehabilitation and Alan Abrams of Far West Laboratories in San Francisco.
127. from a phone interview and personal correspondence with Tapper in 1996.
128. "Is God Listening," *Newsweek*, March 31, 1997, p. 57.
129. ibid. p. 59.
130. Larry Dossey, M.D., *Healing Words: The Power of Prayer and the Practice of Medicine*, San Francisco: Harper, 1993, p. 2.
131. *Brain/Mind Bulletin*, Vol. II #7. Original study is Randolph C. Byrd, "Positive Therapeutic Effects of Intercessory Prayer in a Coronary Care Unit Population," *Southern Medical Journal*, July 1988, Vol. 81 #7, p. 826-29.
132. Larry Dossey, M.D., *Healing Words*, pg. 180.
133. personal interview with Ruzga in 1997.
134. speaking on "Healing and Judaism," co-sponsored by Fairfield County, Connecticut congregations Beth El and B'nai Israel, March, 1997.
135. Justin Stone, *Meditation For Healing*, New Mexico: Sun Books, 1977, p. 86-87.
136. Adapted from Ron DelBene,*The Breath of Life: A Simple Way to Pray*, Upper Room Books, 1992.

Chapter 13
137. *Mental Medicine Update* newsletter, Fall 1993, pg. 7.
138. from a personal interview with Nehlsen in 1995.
139. *Brain/Mind Bulletin*, Vol. IV, Themepack #4, 1979.
140. ibid.
141. *Brain/Mind Bulletin*, Vol. XI, Themepack #5, 1987.
142. ibid.
143. ibid.
144. *Brain/Mind Bulletin*, Vol. VII, Themepack #7, 1982.
145. during a personal interview with Esselstyn in 1984; he continues to do well as we go to press for this new edition.
146. during a personal interview with Dr. Miller in 1984.
147. *Mind/Body Health Newsletter*, 1996, Vol. V #2, p. 3, from an article on preparing for surgery by David Sobel, M.D., and Robert Ornstein, Ph.D.
148. *Health Journeys: Network News*, Issue 4, Naparstek, B., letter from Belleruth, and Research desk, p.1, 1996.
149. during a phone interview with office staff at *Health Journeys* in January, 1997.
150. ibid.

151. from personal interviews with Linda Zelizer in 1983-84
152. *Brain/Mind Bulletin*, May 1988, Vol. XIII #8, p. 2.
153. ibid.
154. from personal correspondence with Tager in February, 1997.
155. from an interview with Tager in 1984; her husband is an M.D., a urologist.

Chapter 14
156. from a personal interview and written correspondence with Dr. Ullman in 1984.
157. *Brain/Mind Bulletin*, 1977, Vol. I & II.
158. ibid.
159. Dr. Stephen Aizenstat in the interview "How to Use Dreams," *Privileged Information* newsletter, March 1989, Vol. 5, #6.
160. This material was first published in *Dream Network Bulletin*.

Chapter 15
161. from personal interviews and correspondence with Thau in 1983-84.
162. ibid.
163. from personal correspondence with Lang in 1984.
164. *Brain/Mind Bulletin*, May 1988, Vol. XIII #8, p. 2.
165. from personal interviews and correspondence with Zelizer in 1983-84.
166. from personal interviews and correspondence with Tager in 1983-84.
167. Jacqui Bishop and Mary Grunte, *How To Forgive When You Don't Know How*, Station Hill Press, 1993, p. 65.
168. ibid.
169. ibid.

Chapter 16
170. Aryeh Kaplan, *Jewish Meditation: A Practical Guide*, Schocken Books, 1985, p. 87.

Recommended Reading

Auw, Andre, Ph.D., *Gentle Roads To Survival: Making Self-Healing Choices in Difficult Circumstances*. Fairfield, CT: Aslan Publishing, 1991.

Auw, Andre, PhD., *The Gift Of Wounding: Finding Hope and Heart in Challenging Circumstances*. Fairfield, CT: Aslan Publishing, 1999.

Advances: The Journal for Mind/Body Health. New York: Institute for Advancement of Health.

American Brain Tumor Association. *A Primer of Brain Tumors: A Patient's Reference Manual*.
2720 River Road, Des Plaines, IL 60018-4110.

American International Reiki Association.. *The Reiki Journal*. 2210 Wilshire Blvd., Suite 831, Santa Monica, CA 90403.

Atkins, Dr. Robert. *Dr. Atkins' Health Revolution: How Complementary Medicine can Extend Your Life*. New York: Houghton-Mifflin, 1988

Bird, Christopher and Tompkins, Peter. *The Secret Life of Plants*. New York: Harper and Row, 1973.

Bishop, Jacqui, M.S. and Grunte, Mary, R.N.. *How to Forgive When You Don't Know How*. New York: Station Hill Press, 1993.

Blythe, Peter. *Self-Hypnotism: Its Power and Practice*. Ontario, Canada: Coles Publishing Co., 1978.

Bondi, Julia A. *Lovelight: Unveiling the Mysteries of Sex and Romance*. New York: Pocket Books, 1989.

Borysenko, Joan, Ph.D. *Minding the Body, Mending the Mind*. New York: Bantam, 1988.

Brown, Barbara B., Ph.D. *Super Mind: The Ultimate Energy*. New York: Harper & Row, 1980

Bruce, Shelly. *Tomorrow is Today*. Indianapolis: Bobbs-Merrill, 1983.

Bryan, Nancy, Ph.D., *Thin Is A State Of Mind*. Minneapolis:CompCare Publications, 1980.

Chapman, Joyce. *If I Had Three Wishes, the Only One Would Be*. North Hollywood, CA: Newcastle Publishing, 1995.

Childre, Doc Lew. *Cut-Thru: A Scientifically Proven Insight on How to Care Without Becoming a Victim*. Boulder Creek, CA: Planetary Publications, 1995.

Childre, Doc Lew. *Freeze Frame: Fast Action Stress Relief* . Boulder Creek, CA: Planetary Publications, 1994.

Church, Dawson. *Communing With the Spirit of Your Unborn Child*. Fairfield, CT: Aslan Publishing, 1988.

Church, Dawson and Sherr, Dr. Alan. *The Heart of the Healer*. Fairfield, CT: Aslan Publishing, 1988.

Cousins, Norman. *Anatomy of an Illness as Perceived by the Patient.* New York: W.W. Norton, 1979.

Cousins, Norman. *The Healing Heart: Antidotes to Panic and Helplessness,* New York: W.W. Norton, 1983.

Desowitz, Robert S., Ph.D. *The Thorn in the Starfish: The Immune System & How it Works.* New York: W. W. Norton, 1987.

Dossey, Larry M.D. *Healing Words: The Power of Prayer and the Practice of Medicine.* New York: HarperCollins, 1993.

Dream Network Bulletin. 670 East Rio Rd., Charlottesville VA 22901.

Egan, Gerard. "Logos: Man's Translation of Himself into Language" in Joseph DeVito, *Language: Concept and Processes.* Englewood Cliffs, NJ: Prentice-Hall, 1973.

Ellenberg, Daniel, Ph.D. & Bell, Judith, M.S., M.F.C.C. *Lovers For Life: Creating Lasting Passion, Trust and True Partnership.* Fairfield, CT: Aslan Publishing, 1995.

Evans, Mike. *The Return.* New York: Thomas Nelson, 1986.

Falcon, Rabbi Ted, Ph.D. *A Journey of Awakening: 49 Steps from Enslavement to Freedom. Skynear Press, PO Box 51241, Seattle, WA 98115, 1999.*

Ferguson, Marilyn. *Brain/Mind Bulletin.* Box 211, Los Angeles, CA 90042.

Ferguson, Marilyn. *The Aquarian Conspiracy: Personal and Social Transformation in the 1980's.* New York: J.P. Tarcher, 1987.

Foundation For Inner Peace. *A Course in Miracles.* PO Box 635, Tiburon, CA 94920,1975.

Frankl, Viktor B. *Man's Search For Meaning: An Introduction To Logotherapy.* New York: Simon & Schuster, 1985.

Freeman, Joel. *God Is Not Fair: Coming to Terms with Life's Raw Deals.* PO Box 1576, San Bernadino, CA 92402, 1987.

Fuller, Elizabeth. *The Touch of Grace.* New York: Dodd, Mead, 1986.

Friedlander, Mark and Phillips, Terry. *Winning the War Within.* Emmaus, PA: Rodale Press, 1986.

Gawain, Shakti. *Creative Visualization.* Mill Valley, CA: New World Library, 1978.

Gerson, Max, M.D. *A Cancer Therapy.* PO Box 1035, Del Mar, CA 92014: Totality Books, 1975.

Glasser, Ronald J., M.D. *The Body Is the Hero.* New York: Random House, 1976.

Glasser, William. *Positive Addiction.* New York: Harper & Row, 1976.

Goleman, Daniel. *The Varieties of the Meditative Experience.* New York: Irvington, 1977.

Goleman, Daniel. *Vital Lies, Simple Truths: The Psychology of Self-Deception*. New York: Simon and Schuster, 1985.

Goleman, Daniel & Guerin, Joel, Editors. *Mind Body Medicine: How to Use Your Mind For Better Health*. Yonkers, New York: Consumer Reports Books, 1993.

Green, Lila. *Making Sense of Humor: How to Add Joy to Your Life*. KIT Publishing 1131 Tolland Tkpe., Suite 175, Manchester, CT 06040, 1994.

Gress, Barbara J., *Personal Power Cards™, Flashcards For Emotional Wellness*. Blue Topaz Publishing, P.O. Box 480, Mount Shasta, CA 96067, 1991.

Harms, Valerie. *The Inner Lover: Using Passion as a Way to Self-Empowerment*. Fairfield, CT: Aslan Publishing, 1999.

Halacy, D.S. *Man and Memory: Breakthroughs in the Science of the Human Mind*. New York: Harper & Row, 1970.

Halpern, Steven, Ph.D. *Tuning the Human Instrument*. 1775 Old Country Road, #19, Belmont, CA 94002: Spectrum Research Institute, 1978.

Hay, Louise L. *You Can Heal Your Life*. Carlsbad, CA: Hay House Inc. 1987.

Hendrickson, Peter A. *Alive & Well: A Path For Living in a Time of HIV*. New York: Irvington Publishers, 1990.

Hunt, Morton. *The Universe Within: A New Science Explores the Human Mind*. New York: Simon and Schuster, 1982.

Hirshberg,Caryle & Barasch, Marc Ian. *Remarkable Recovery: What Extraordinary Healings Tell us About Getting Well and Staying Well*. New York: Riverhead Books/ G.P. Putnam, 1995.

Jaffe, Dennis T., Ph.D. *Healing From Within*. New York: Alfred Knopf, 1980.

Janiger, Oscar, M.D. & Goldberg, Philip. *A Different Kind of Healing: Doctors Speak Candidly About Their Successes with Alternative Medicine*. New York: Tarcher/Putnam, 1993.

Johnson, Judi & Klein, Linda. *I Can Cope: Stay Healthy with Cancer.* P.O. Box 47945, Minneapolis, MN 55447: Chronimed Publishing, 1994.

Kabat-Zinn, Jon, Ph.D. *Wherever You Go, There You Are: Mindfulness Meditation in Everyday Life*. New York: Hyperion, 1994.

Kaplan, Aryeh. *Jewish Meditation: A Practical Guide*. New York: Schocken Books, 1985.

Katz, Alice, M.S. *It's Not Personal: A Guide to Anger Management*. Westport, CT: AJK Publishing, 1996.

King, Lester S. *The Growth of Medical Thought*. Chicago: University of Chicago Press, 1963.

Koestler, Arthur. *The Lotus and the Robot.* New York: Macmillan, 1961.

Koestler, Arthur. *The Ghost in the Machine.* New York: Macmillan, 1967.

Kornfield, Jack with Gil Fronsdal. *Teachings of the Buddha.* Boston: Shambhala,1993.

Lance, James W. *Headache: Understanding Alleviation.* New York: Scribners, 1975.

LeCron, Leslie M. *Self-Hypnotism.* New York: New American Library, 1964.

Lewis, Howard R. and Martha E. *Psychosomatics: How Your Emotions Can Damage Your Health.* New York: Viking, 1972.

Lynch, James J. *The Broken Heart: The Medical Consequences of Loneliness.* New York: Basic Books, 1977.

Miller, Emmett, M.D., and Lueth, Deborah, Ph.D. *Self Imagery.* Berkeley: Celestial Arts, 1986.

Monte, Tom and the editors of East West Natural Health. *World Medicine: The East West Guide to Healing Your Body.* New York: Tarcher/Putnam, 1993.

Nehlsen, Nancy and Stewart, Marjabelle. *Princess Marjabelle Visits Lollygag Lake.* Fairfield, CT: Robert B. Luce, 1996.

Northrup, Christiane, M.D. *Women's Bodies, Women's Wisdom.* New York: Bantam 1994;

Pearsall, Paul, Ph.D. *Superimmunity: Master Your Emotions and Improve Your Health.* New York: McGraw-Hill, 1987.

Pelletier, Kenneth. *Mind as Healer, Mind as Slayer.* New York: Dell, 2nd. ed., 1992.

Perkins, William. *Moving to the Positive Side.* Lima, Ohio: Fairway Press, 1992.

Postman, Neil. *Crazy Talk, Stupid Talk.* New York: Delacorte Press, 1976.

Rainer, Tristine. *The New Diary.* Los Angeles: J.P. Tarcher, 1978.

Radha, Swami Sivananda. *Seeds of Light.* Box 160, Porthill, ID 83853: Timeless Books, 1985.

Reed, Henry. *Dream Realizations: A Dream Incubation Workbook.* 503 Lake Drive, Virginia Beach, VA 23451, 1984.

Reuben, Carolyn. "Aids: The Promise of Alternative Treatments," pp. 52–66. *East West Journal.* Sept., 1986.

Rodegast, Pat and Stanton, Judith. *Emmanuel's Book: A Manual for Living Comfortably in the Cosmos.* New York: Bantam Books, 1994.

Roger, John and McWilliams, Peter. *You Can't Afford the Luxury of a Negative Thought.* Box 69773, Los Angeles, CA 90069: Prelude Press, 1988.

Rosanoff, Nancy. *Intuition Workout: A Practical Guide to Discovering and Developing Your Inner Knowing, 2nd ed.* Fairfield, CT: Aslan Publishing, 1991.

Rosenbaum, Jean M.D. *The Mind Factor: How Your Emotions Affect Your Health.* Englewood Cliffs, NJ: Prentice-Hall, 1973.

Rosman, Rabbi Steven M. *Deena the Damselfly*, New York: UAHC Press, 1992.

Rosman, Rabbi Steven M. *Spiritual Parenting*, Wheaton, IL: Quest Books, 1994.

Rosman, Rabbi Steven M., Ph.D., M.S *Jewish Healing Wisdom,* Northvale, NJ: Jason Aronson Inc. , 1997.

Sarno, John E. M.D. *Healing Back Pain—The Mind-Body Connection.* New York: Warner Books, 1991

Schloff, Laurie & Yudkin, Marcia. *Smart Speaking.* New York: Plume, 1991.

Schloff, Laurie & Yudkin, Marcia. *He & She Talk.* New York: Plume, 1993.

Siegel, Bernie S., M.D. *Love, Medicine & Miracles.* New York: Harper & Row, 1986.

Siegel, Bernie S., M.D. *Peace, Love & Healing.* New York: Harper & Row, 1989.

Siegel, Bernie S., M.D. *How to Live Between Office Visits.* New York: HarperCollins, 1993.

Siegel, Bernie S., M.D. *Prescriptions for Living: Inspirational Lessons For a Joyful, Loving Life.* New York: HarperCollins, 1998.

Silva, Jose. *The Silva Mind Control Method.* Pocket Books, 1977.

Simonton, Carl. *Getting Well Again: A Step by Step Self-Help Guide to Overcoming Cancer for Patients and Their Families.* Los Angeles: J.P. Tarcher, 1978.

Smithsonian Magazine. 900 Jefferson Drive, Washington, DC 20560.

Sontag, Susan. *Illness as Metaphor.* New York: Farrar, Straus & Giroux, 1977.

Steincrohn, Peter J., M.D. and LaFia, David, M.D. *How to Master Your Nerves.* New York: Cowles, 1970.

Stocking, Jerry. *Cognitive Harmony: An Adventure in Mental Fitness.* P.O. Box 335, Chetek, WI 54728: Moose Ear Press. 1991.

Stone, Christopher. *Re-Creating Your Self.* P.O. Box 10616, Portland, OR 97210: Metamorphous Press.

Stone, Justin F. *Meditation For Healing!* P.O. Box 4383, Albuquerque, NM 87106: Sun Publishing, 1977.

Ullman, Montague, M.D. and Zimmerman, Nan. *Working With Dreams.* Los Angeles: J.P. Tarcher, 1979.

Ullman, Montague, M.D. and Linner, Claire. *The Variety of Dream Experience.* New York: Continuum Publishers, 1987.

Vlahos, Olivia. *Body: The Ultimate Symbol.* New York: Lippincott, 1979.

Wallace, Amy and Henkin, Bill. *The Psychic Healing Book.* New York: Dell, 1978.

Ward, Milton. *The Brilliant Function of Pain.* NY: Optimus Books, c/o CSA Press, Lakemont, GA, 1977.

Weil, Andrew, M.D. *Natural Health, Natural Medicine.* Boston: Houghton-Mifflin, 1990.

Westlake, Aubrey T. *The Pattern of Health.* Berkeley: Shambhala, 1973.

Wooten, Patty, R.N. *Compassionate Laughter: Jest For Your Health.* P.O.Box 58673, Salt Lake City, UT 84158: Commune-a-Key Publishing, 1996.

Wylen, Rabbi Stephen M. *Gossip: The Power of the Word.* Hoboken, NJ, KTAV Publishing House, Inc. 1993.

Resources: Individuals

The following is a sampling of the many resources available to you. Included are the addresses and/or phone numbers and websites of many of the health professionals and others who contributed to this book Inclusion on this resource list is not meant as a blanket endorsement. It just means that I believe they have something of value to share.

Jacqui Bishop and **Mary Grunte**,
authors and workshop leaders
Box 97, Bronxville, NY 10708
Bishop: 914-997-9611
jbishop@bestweb.net
Grunte: 914-793-6418; 914-684-1860 Fax

Mark A. Breiner, D.D.S., author,
Whole Body Dentistry
5520 Park Ave., Trumbull, CT 06611
203-371-0300
www.wholebodydentistry.com
Mercury-free holistic dentistry

Adam Breiner, N.D., Naturopath
Whole Body Medicine
5520 Park Ave., Trumbull, CT 06611
203-371-8258
www.wholebodymed.com
Holistic healthcare

Brian Baker, D.C., Chiropractor
133 Reef Rd , Fairfield, CT 06824
203-259-5836
reefchirocare@snet.net

Harry Brown, M.D.
Weston, CT, 203-226-6670
Psychiatrist

Rosalyn Bruyere, founder,
Healing Light Center Church
261 E. Alegria Ave. #12, Sierra Madre, CA 91024; 626-306-2170, 626-355-0996 Fax
www.rosalynlbruyere org
hlcc2@earthlink.net
A unique comprehensive training program on healing.

Robert Burd, M.D.
Medical Specialists of Fairfield
425 Post Road, Fairfield, CT 06824
203-255-4545
Oncology, Hematology, Internal Medicine

David Bushell, M.D.
501 Kings Highway East
Fairfield, CT 06825
203-610-6300
Internal and Pulmonary Medicine

Judy Chessin, APRN, MNS,
162 Toilsome Hill Rd, Fairfield, CT 06825
203-949-4412
Compassionate Nursing

Michael Dogali, M.D.,
USC Neurosurgery and Neurology
1510 San Pablo St # 268, Los Angeles, CA 90033
323-442-1799 or 323-442-5720
The neurosurgeon who performed my brain surgery (bhi)

Wallace C. Ellerbroek, M.D. (deceased)
Anyone interested in a more technical, in-depth understanding of Dr. Ellerbroek's treatment program can read "Language Thought and Disease" in *Perspectives in Biology and Medicine*, Vol 16, No 2, Winter 1973 A simpler version appears as "Language, Thought and Disease" in *Co-Evolution Quarterly*, No 17, Spring 1978.

Erik Esselstyn, President
Cross Creek Initiative (CCI)
www chesapeake.net/dh/CCI html
esselstyn@aol.com
Nonprofit organization "to champion the worldwide shift to maximum efficiency and planet-friendly energy."

Rabbi Ted Falcon, Ph.D.
Rabbi@betalef org
206-522-7399
Bet Alef Meditational Synagogue
PO Box 51049, Seattle, WA 98115-1049
206-527-9399 • www betalef org
Rabbi Ted Falcon is a practicing psychotherapist, congregational rabbi, author and teacher who regularly conducts workshops and retreats.

John Graham, Executive Director
The Giraffe Project
Box 759, Langley, WA 98260
www giraffe.org • office@giraffe org
"Moving people to stick their necks out for the common good."

Barbara J. Gress (Semple)
PO Box 480, Mount Shasta, CA 96067
530-926-0804
Private practice offering psycho-spiritual
support using her *Personal Power
Cards™— Flashcards For Emotional
Wellness* and Jin Shin Jyutsu(r), an Oriental
energy healing art.

Carl Gruning, O.D.
Eye Care Associates
2600 Post Road, Fairfield, CT 06824
203-255-4005; 203-259-8748 Fax
Behavioral Optometrist; Vision therapy

Louise Hay, author and lecturer
Hay House, Inc.
P.O Box 5100, Carlsbad, CA. 92018
Books and tapes: 1-800-654 5126
Fax orders 1-800-650 5115
www.hayhouse.com

Steve Hirshorn, M.D.
2660 Main St., Suite 302
Bridgeport, CT 06606
203-331-8700, 203-335-5819 Fax
Colon and Rectal Surgery

Alice Katz, artist and therapist
296 Partridge Lane, Fairfield, CT 06824
203-259-8026
Alice@GoodLivingBooks com
www.GoodLivingBooks com
Author, anger management and compulsive
eating issues

Steven Kunkes, M.D.
1305 Post Road, Fairfield, CT 06480
203-292-2000; 203-292-0804 Fax
Cardiologist

Bob Lang, M.D
60 Washington Ave , Suite 105
Hamden, CT. 06518
203-248-4362; 203-248-6933 Fax
Endocrinologist, Internist; Healing conversations

Richard Levin, M.D., D.M.D.
1305 Post Road, Fairfield, CT 06480
203-259-4700
Otolaryngology; Ear, Nose and Throat

Kenneth Lipow, M.D., Neurosurgeon
CT Neurosurgical Specialists
267 Grant St , Bridgeport, CT 06610
203-384-4500

Dr. James T. De Villamil Long, N.D.
D.D., holistic counselor
1-888-337-0511 for telephone consultations
www.naturalhealthinfo.com
www.spiritualhealth.com
info@longnaturalhealth com

Robert A Marshall, D.C., Chiropractor
40 Red Coat Road, Westport, CT 06880
203-226-6366

Emmett Miller, M.D , author & radio host,
Source Cassettes (guided imagery)
131 East Placer St., Auburn, CA 95604
530-478-1807, 800-528-2737 Toll-free
800-882-1840 Toll-free fax
www.drmiller com • drmiller@drmiller com
California Task Force on Self-Esteem,
founder and medical director of The Cancer
Support and Education Center in Menlo
Park, California

Rabbi Goldie Milgram
Reclaiming Judaism as a Spiritual Practice
http //www.rebgoldie.com

Belleruth Naparstek, LISW, Health
Journeys, Image Paths, Inc ,
891 Moe Drive Ste C, Akron, OH 44310
800-800-8661 Toll-free, 330-633-3831
www.healthjourneys.com
info@healthjourneys com • hjtapes@aol.com
Network News, a free quarterly newsletter
of studies, reviews & inspiring stories

Randall H. Neichen, D.M.D.,
Periodontist
4699 Main St., Bridgeport, CT 06606
203-372-3575

Christiane Northrup, M.D.,
Past President
American Holistic Medical Association
PO Box 199, Yarmouth, Maine 04096
www. DrNorthrup com
Call 1-800-804-0935 to subscribe to her
newsletter *Health Wisdom for Women.*
There is a monthly message hotline for
subscribers only.

Larry Novik, M.D.
698 Brooklawn Ave., Bridgeport, CT 06604
203-366-1288

Buryl Payne, Ph.D., Psycho Physics Labs
1803 Mission St Suite 24
Santa Cruz, CA 95060
831-462-1588 • www.buryl.com
books and tapes, magnetic instruments

Nancy Rosanoff, *Intuition Workout*
Author/lecturer
914-769-7226;
Website: www intuitionatwork.com

**Rabbi Steven M. Rosman, L.Ac., Ph.D.,
M.S.**, Acupuncture, Oriental Medicine,
Nutrition; Director, Division of Complementary Medicine, Prohealth Care Associates
2 ProHealth Plaza
Lake Success, NY 11042
516-608-2880, 516-883-5811 Fax
Author of *Jewish Healing Wisdom* and
Spiritual Parenting

Jacqueline Ruzga, D.C , Chiropractor
2452 Black Rock Turnpike,
Fairfield, CT 06825
203-372-7333; 203-372-1348 Fax

Dr. John Sarno, M.D.
author, *Healing Back Pain*
Howard Rusk Institute of Rehabilitation
Medicine
400 East 34th St., NYC 10016
212-263-6035 office
212-263-7300 Rusk Institute
www.med.nyu.edu

Marvin Schweitzer, N.D , Naturopath
Wellness Institute
1 Westport Ave., Norwalk, CT 06851
203 -847-2788, 203-847 2739 Fax
www.wellnessinstitute-ct.com

Robban Sica, M.D., Medical Director,
Center for the Healing Arts, PC
370 Post Rd , Orange, Ct 06477
203-799-7733; 203-799-3560 Fax
www.centerhealingarts org

Bernie Siegel, M.D.
Fax 203 387 8355
www.drbernie.com bugsysiegel@cs com
author and lecturer, purchase tapes c/o Hay
House, Inc., 1-800-654-5126
1-800-650-5115 Fax orders only

Elizabeth Spark, M.D.
1400 Centre St., Suite 105, Newton
Centre, MA 02459
781-235-6444, 617-630-0601 Fax
Behavioral medicine; hypnotherapy

Roberta K. Tager, M.S.
104 Imperial Ave., Westport, CT 06880
203-226-4548 or 561-691-3233
Health counseling and therapy

David A. Tapper
P. O. Box 900, Woodstock,
New York 12498

Barry Taylor, N.D., Naturopath,
New England Family Health Center
270 Winter Street, Weston, MA 02493
781-237-8505

Dorothy Thau
0536 Meadowood Drive
Aspen, Colorado 81611
970-925-6621, 970-920-2209 Fax
thau@aspeninfo com
Holistic health counselor/parapsychologist

Professor Montague Ullman, M.D.
55 Orlando Ave , Ardsley, N Y 10502
914-693-0156; 914-693-3942 Fax
Psychoanalyst & author; dream workshops

Marianne Williamson, author and lecturer
c/o Hay House, Inc.
P.O. Box 5100, Carlsbad, CA 92018
Books and tapes: 1-800-654-5126
www Marianne com

Linda Zelizer, Hypnotherapist,
Center For Personal Development
P.O. BOX 1134, Woodstock, NY 12498
845-679-0813 • zelizer@banet.net
Workshops; private practice; consultant to
business on human relations skills.

Resources: Organizations

The Academy for Jewish Religion
6301 Riverdale Ave., Riverdale, NY10471
718-543-3700; 7180543-1038 Fax;
www arjsem org

Acoustic Neuroma Association (ANA)
600 Peachtree Parkway, Suite 108
Cummings, GA 30041-6899
770-205-8211, 770-205-0239 Fax
www.anausa org • info@anausa.org
Support for brain tumor patients, newsletter

ALEPH: Alliance For Jewish Renewal
Debra Kolodny, Executive Director
7000 Lincoln Drive, #82,
Philadelphia, PA 19119-3048
215-247-0210
www.aleph org • alephajr@aol com
Programs/resources/networks for groups
and individuals involved in Jewishy renewal,
send for membership packet, quarterly
journal, *New Menorah*

American Brain Tumor Association (ABTA)
2720 River Road, Des Plaines, IL 60018-4110
847-827-9910; 847-827-9918 Fax
1-800-886-2282 Patient line
www.abta.org • info@abta.org
Patient education; research

American Chiropractic Association
1701 Clarendon Blvd.
Arlington, VA 22209
800-986-4636; 703-243-2593 Fax
www.amerchiro.org
memberinfo@amerchiro.org

American Chronic Pain Association (ACPA)
P.O. Box 850, Rocklin, CA 95677
916-632-0922; 916-632-3208 Fax
www.theacpa.org • acpa@pacbell.net

American Holistic Medical Association
12101 Menaul Blvd. NE, Suite C
Albuquerque, NM 87112
Lawrence B. Palevsky, M.D., President
505-292-7788; 505-293-7582 Fax
www.holisticmedicine.org
"Holistic Medicine is the Art and Science of
healing that addresses the whole person
Body, Mind and Spirit"

American Holistic Nurses Association
P.O. Box 2130, Flagstaff, AZ 86003-2130
800-278-2462, www.ahna.org
info@ahna.org

American Institute Of Stress
Dr. Paul J. Rosch President
124 Park Ave, Yonkers, NY 10703
914-963-1200, 914-965-6267 Fax:
www.stress.org • stress124@opton.net

American Music Therapy Association
8455 Colesville Rd., Ste 1000,
Silver Spring, MD 20910
301-589-5175, www.musictherapy.org
info@musictherapy.org

American Polarity Therapy Association
2888 Bluff St., Ste 149
Boulder, CO 80301
800-359-5620l; www.polaritytherapy.org

The American Society Of Hypertension (ASH)
148 Madison Ave., 5th floor
New York, NY 10016
212-644-0650; 212-644-0658 Fax
www.ash-us.org • ash@ash-us.org
Scientific organization for education,
research and treatment strategies devoted
exclusively to hypertension and related
cardiovascular diseases.

Association for Applied Psychophysiology and Biofeedback
10200 W. 44th Avenue, Ste 304,
Wheat Ridge, CO 80033-2840
800-477-8892 Toll-free; 303-422-8436
www.aapb.org • AAPB@resourcenter.com
For informationn packet and practitioners
list send SASE via snail mail.

Association For Research And Enlightenment (ARE)
The Edgar Cayce Foundation
215 67th St., Virginia Beach, VA 23451
Info: 1-800-333-4499
Books and Tapes· 1-800-723-1112
757-422-6921 Fax • www.are-cayce.com

Brain/Mind Institute and ***Bulletin***
Marilyn Ferguson, Founder & Publisher
4047 San Rafael Ave.
Los Angeles, CA 90065
MLferg@earthlink.net
Send SASE for information on available
collections of articles; Marilyn Ferguson is
interested in hearing from readers about
their personal experiences which corroborate or illustrate the principles in *Your Body
Believes Every Word You Say.*

Buddhism Information Network— Gateway to Buddhism
www.buddhanet.net
Information on various Buddhist traditions.

Central Brain Tumor Registry of the United States (CBTRUS)
244 East Ogdenn Ave., Suite 116
Hinsdale, IL 60521
630-655-4786, 630-655-4756 Fax
www.cbtrus.org • cbtrus@aol.com
Collects and disseminates high quality
incidence data on all primary brain tumors.

**Congregation B'nai Israel,
Rabbi James Prosnit**
2710 Park Ave, Bridgeport, CT 06604
203-336-1858
www.congregationbnaiisrael.org

The Cooper Aerobics Center
12200 Preston Road, Dallas, TX 75230
1-800-444-5764 or 972-239-7223
972-239-6649 Fax
www.cooperaerobics.com

The Counseling Center
Sarah Gewanter MSW, LCSW, and
Denny Cooper
7 Tokeneke Road; Darien CT 06820
203-655-1091; 203 656 4556 Fax
www.vision3d.com/adhd
gewanter@aol.com
Psychotherapy, hypnotherapy, meditation,
stress reduction and Auditory Integration
Training (AIT) for ADD/ADHD, CAPD,
PDD and Autism

Elat Chayyim
A Center For Healing And Renewal
99 Mill Hook Road, Accord, NY 12404
800-398-2630; 845-626-0157
845-626-2037 Fax
www.elatchayyim org
generalinfo@elatchayyim.org
Transdenominational Jewish spiritual retreat
and workshop center

Esalen Institute
Highway 1, Big Sur, CA 93920
831-667-3000, 831-667-2724 Fax
www.esalen.org • info@esalen org
Holistic retreat/alternative education center

Fetzer Institute
9292 West KL Ave., Kalamazoo, MI 49009
616-375-2000; 616-372-2163 Fax
www.fetzer org • info@fetzer.org
Supports research, education and service
programs on mind/body/spirit health;
*Advances: The Journal for Mind-Body
Health*

**Foundation For Advancement in
Cancer Therapy (FACT)**
Ruth Sackman, President
P.O. Box 1242, Old Chelsea Station,
New York, NY 10113
212-741-2790; www.Fact-Ltd.org
Clearinghouse for information on biologically
sound alternative cancer therapies, lifestyle
changes

Gerson Institute
1572 Second Ave., San Diego, CA 92101
619-685-5353
www.gerson.org • info@gerson org
Nutrition and detoxification to heal cancer
and chronic and degenerative disease

Insight Transformational Seminars and
the **University of Santa Monica**
John-Roger Chancellor USM/Insight
2101 Wilshire Blvd.,
Santa Monica, CA 90403
310-829-7402

Institute of HeartMath (IHM)
Doc Lew Childre, Founder and President
P O. Box 1463 Boulder Creek, CA 95006
831-338-8500
www heartmath.org • info@heartmath.org
Training and research into role of heart in
human intelligence and health.

Institute of Noetic Sciences
101 San Antonio Rd , Petaluma, CA 94952
707-775-3500, 707-781-7420 Fax
www noetic.org
Education and research in human consciousness

**International Imagery Association &
Image Institute**
Akhter Ahsen, Founding Chairman
22 Edgecliff Terrace, Yonkers, NY 10705
914-423-5291 or 914-423-9200
914-376-3671 Fax; ahsena@aol.com
Eidetic Image-Based Therapy; information
and training, allergy relief.

**Internationational Institute of Reflexol-
ogy**
P O. Box 12642, St Petersburg, FL 33733
813-343-4811

**International Mahavir Jain Mission—
Siddhachalam**
65 Mud Pond Road; Blairstown, NJ 07825
908-362-9793; 908-362-9649 Fax
www.imjm org
Programs in Jain philosphy, non-violence,
healing, chanting.

**International Medical and Dental
Hypnotherapy Association (IMDHA)**
4110 Edgeland Ave, Ste 800,
Royal Oak, MI 48073-2285
248-549-5594, 800-257-5467 Toll-free
www.infinityinst.com
aspencer@infinityinst.com
Referral service of certified hypnotherapists

International Network for Attitudinal Healing
Jerry Jampolsky M.D., Founder,
Trish Ellis, Executive Director
33 Buchanan Drive, Sausalito, CA 94965
888-222-7205 Toll-free
415-331-6161 X111, 415-331-4545 Fax
www.attitudinalhealing.org
www healingcenter.org

International Society For the Study of Subtle Energies and Energy Medicine (ISSSEEM)
356 Goldco Circle,
Golden, CO 80403-1347
303-425-4625; 303-425-4685 Fax
www. Nekesc.org /~issseem/
issseem@compuserve.com
Interdisciplinary membership

Islam: Muslim Information
Imam Nasif Muhammad, Mosjia Al Aziz
Temple: 203-368-3766 in CT
Imam W. D. Mohammed
www.worldforum.com/islam.htm

Kripalu Center For Yoga And Health
P.O Box 793, Lenox, MA 01240
West State Route 183
800-741-7353; www kripalu.org
Retreat and workshops. yoga, self-discovery, spiritual attunement and holistic health

The Miami Project to Cure Paralysis
P.O. Box 016960, R-48 PPW,
Miami, FL 33101
305-243-6001; 305-243-6017 Fax
www miamiproject.miami.edu
Research on spinal cord injuries, patient information

Mid Fairfield AIDS Project
16 River St., Norwalk, CT 06850
203-865-9535
www.mfap.com (links with other AIDS sites)

Naropa University (Buddhist based)
2130 Arapahoe Ave., Boulder, CO 80302
303-444-0202 admissions; 303-346-3504
on line classes; www.naropa edu
Accredited degree programs based on Buddhist educational heritage and philosophy; non-degree school of continuing ed

National Alliance for the Mentally Ill (NAMI)
Colonial Place Three
2107 Wilson Blvd., Suite 300
Arlington, VA 22201-3042
1-800-950-6264 Toll-free
www.nami.org • helpline@nami.org
Grass roots self-help organization dedicated to improving the lives of people with severe, biologically-based brain disorders

The National Center For Jewish Healing
850 7th Ave., New York, NY 10019
212-399-2320; 212-399-2475 Fax;
www.jbfcs.org
Newsletter,*The Outstretched Arm*;
educational programs.

National Foundation for Brain Research & National Coalition for Research in Neurological Disorders
1250 24th St. NW, Ste. 300, Washington DC 20037
202-293-5453, 202-466-0585 Fax
www brainnet org
Conferences on neurological research and emerging treatments

National HIV/AIDS Hotline
AM Social Health Association
P.O. Box 13821, Research Triangle PK, NC 27709
919-361-8400; 919-361-8425 Fax
www ashastd org
General information and referrals

National Institute For the Clinical Application of Behavioral Medicine (NICABM)
P.O. Box 523, Mansfield Center, CT 06250
1-800-743-2226, 860-423-4512 Fax
www nicabm.com • nicabm@neca.com
Conferences for healing professionals and others in mind-body therapies;
audio tapes and workbooks available

National Institute of Mental Health (NIMH)
6001 Executive Boulevard, Rm. 8184,
MSC 9663,
Bethesda, MD 20892-9663
301-443-4513; 866-615-6464 Toll-free
www.nimh.nih.gov • nimhinfo@nih.gov

National Women's Health Network
514 Tenth St. NW, Ste 400
Washington DC 20004
202-347-1140; 202-347-1168
Membership organization; *Network News*
provides women's health information.

New York Open Center
83 Spring St , New York, NY 10012
212-219-2527; 212-219-1347
www.opencenter.org
Holistic healing classes

Obsessive-Compulsive and other bio-chemical Disorders (OC Foundation)
National Headquarters, P.O. Box 70,
Milford, CT 06460-0070
203-878-5669; 203-874-2826 Fax
www ocfoundation.org
info@ocfoundation org

Omega Institute for Holistic Studies
Stephan Rechtschaffen, M.D., Co-founder and President
150 Lake Drive
Rhinebeck, NY 12572-3252
800-944-1001 Toll-free, 845-266-3769
www.eomega.org

The Option Institute
2080 South Undermountain Road,
Sheffield, MA 02157-9643
413-229-2100; 413-229-8931 Fax
www.option.org • happiness@option org

Ozark Research Institute
PO Box 387, Fayetteville, AR 72702-0387
479-582-9197; 479-582-3684 Fax
www.ozarkresearch.org • ori@ipa.net
Research into the power of thought.

Peoples Medical Society,
Charles Inlander, President
462 Walnut Street, Allentown, PA 18102
610-770-1670; 610-770-0607 Fax
www.peoplesmedical org
Consumer advocacy group that also
publishes health-related books.

The Reiki Alliance
P.O. Box 41, Cataldo, ID 83810
208-682-3535

The Rolf Institute
205 Canyon Blvd., Boulder, CO 80302
303-449-5903

Rowe Camp & Conference Center
Kings Highway Road, Rowe, MA 01367
413-339-4954, 413-339-5728 Fax
www.rowecenter.org
Retreat@RoweCenter.org
Workshops year round

Spring Hill Music
Body, Mind & Soul Music
1835 38th St. Ste SW,
Boulder, CO 80301-2605
1-800-427-7860; 303-938-1191 Fax
netcomm@springhillmedia.com
Robert Gass, On Wings Of Song, and more

Sufi Order International/ North
American Secretariat
P.O. Box 30065, Seattle, WA 98103
206-525-6992, 206-525-7013 Fax
www.sufiorder org • sufioffice@aol com

Transpersonal Drama Therapy
Training
Saphira Linden, Penny Lewis & Sarah
Benson, Omega Theater
P O Box 1227, Jamaica Plain, MA 02130
617-522-8300 Phone and Fax
www omegatheater.org • saphiral@aol com

Vestibular Disorders Association
(VEDA)
P.O. Box 13305, Portland, OR 97213
503-229-7705; 800-837-8428 Toll-free
503-229-8064 Fax
www vestibular.org • veda@vestibular.org
For inner-ear balance disorders

Wainwright House
260 Stuyvesant Avenue, Rye, NY 10580
914-967-6080 • www wainwright.org
Oldest nonprofit, nonsectarian holistic
educational center in the United States
where people can find their own paths for
the integration of body, mind and spirit, I
personally spent many rewarding hours here
on retreat or in seminars (bhl)

Wisdom Networks
Life Balance Media LLC (TV, radio, Internet)
10 East 40th Street, 26th floor
New York, NY 10016
304-589-5111 Ext. 1156
www.wisdomnetworks.com
"Programming that can change your life!"

Resources: Prayer

Regardless of your religion you can call or write these groups for prayers

Abundant Life Prayer Group— Oral and Richard Roberts
Tulsa, OK 74171 • 918-495-7777
24 hour prayer line.

Church Of White Eagle Lodge, St. John's Retreat Center
P.O. Box 930, Montgomery, TX 77356
409-597-5757; 409-597-5994 Fax
www.saintjohns.org • sjrc@saintjohns.org

Grace N' Vessels of Christ Ministry
P O Box 3257, Danbury, CT 06813-3257
203-778-hope (4673)
www.gracenvessels.org
24-hour prayer line; prison ministry, newsletter; musical healing services

Jewish Prayers—Online
cholim@torah.org
Email prayer healing list, send patient's Hebrew name and mother's Hebrew name.

Jewish Prayers— Refuah/ Yeshuah
P.O. Box 1212, 1469 42nd St , Brooklyn, NY 11219-9833
24-hour hotline. 1-800-545-PRAY (7729), 718-436-0666; 718-972-2787 Fax
www.refuah.org • ry146942@aol.com
Prayer, personal services and counseling, hotline for prayers at Western Wall in Israel.

Kenneth Copeland Ministries
Fort Worth, TX 76192
800-600-7395 daytime prayer line
www.kcm.org

Mike Evans Ministries
P.O. Box 612128, Dallas, TX 75261-9813

Robert Schuller, Hour of Power
Garden Grove, CA 92840
714-NEW-HOPE (639-4673)
www.newhopeonline.org
24-hr. prayer line; counseling and literature

Silent Unity
1901 NW Blue Parkway
Unity Village, MO 64065
800-669-7729 (24 hour prayer line)
816-524-3550
www.silentunity org; www.unityonline.org
Books and tapes; monthly prayer magazine, *The Daily Word*

Resources: Medical Centers and Hospitals

The following are hospitals where I had surgery or rehabilation related to the brain tumor.

Bridgeport Hospital
267 Grant St., Bridgeport, CT 06610
203-384-3000, 888-833-2220 Toll-free
www.bridgeporthospital.com

Columbia Presbyterian Medical Center—Neurological Institute
622 West 165th St
New York, NY 10032-3784
212-305-2500 • www nyp org

Gaylord Rehabilitation Center
Box 400, Wallingford, CT 06492
Gaylord Farm Road
1-866-429-5673 Toll-free; 203-284-2800
203-284-2700 TDD
www gaylord.org

St. Vincent's Medical Center
2800 Main St , Bridgeport, CT 06606
203-576-6000; 1-877-255-7847 Toll-free
www.stvincents.org

Yale-New Haven Hospital
20 York St., New Haven, CT 06504
203-688-2000 • www ynhh.org
Monthly brain tumor support group. 203-737-1671 or email
elizabeth.dandrea@yale.edu

Index

University of Pittsburgh *232*
upset, meanings of *163*
urinate *144*
urticaria *61*

V

victim *18, 30*
virus *14*
visualization *11, 30, 129, 142, 197*
    exercise *238*
    guidelines *210*

W

walking *182*
Ward, Milton *62*
weight *165, 167*
Weil, Andrew, M.D. *29*
wellness, subjective evaluation of *84*
whiplash *36, 45*
witnessing self *175, 181*
    exercise *102*
witnessing, self *12*
Woldenberg, Lee *218*

Y

Yale Medical Center *9*

Z

Zelizer, Linda
    106, 110, 130, 202, 232

About the Author

Barbara Hoberman Levine was stricken with a large, but slow-growing, brain tumor at the age of 32. After being misdiagnosed for years and undergoing numerous tests, she began looking at the role language played in reinforcing her illness. Her discoveries helped her to recover from the ill-effects of the tumor and the 1985 brain surgery which removed what had become a life-threatening "growth." Instead of crippling or killing her, the "growth" made her stronger and led to this book.

Levine and her husband Harold have three children and two grandchildren. They live in Fairfield, Connecticut.

Contacting the Author

Barbara Hoberman Levine
2490 Black Rock Turnpike, # 342
Fairfield, CT 06825
203-372-0300
203-374-4766 fax
www.wordsworkpress.com

Barbara enjoys hearing from her readers. For a written reply to snail mail, please include a stamped, self-addressed envelope. Barbara is available for counseling and phone consultations. Call or write for an appointment.